HEALTHY DIET FOR SLEEP DISORDERS

An In-depth Dietary Approach to Managing Sleep Disorders, Improving Sleep Quality, and Obtaining Better Health.

Sonia Cline

Copyright 2024 @ Sonia Cline

DISCLAIMER

ABOUT THE AUTHOR

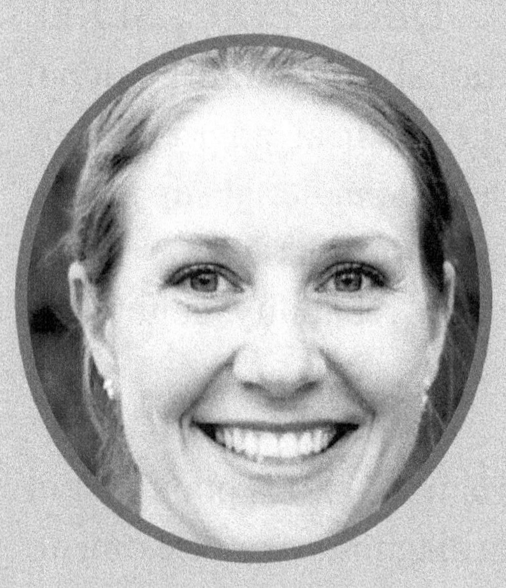 Sonia Cline is a professional chef who is passionate about preparing nutritious and delicious meals that encourage health and well-being. With years of culinary experience, Sonia has dedicated her career to researching the relationship between diet and general health. Her ability to create well-balanced dishes, as well as her dedication to using fresh, healthful products, have earned her reputation in the culinary industry.

Sonia's path into healthy eating began with a goal to enhance her own and her family's health. This personal quest inspired her to research diverse food patterns and their effects on numerous facets of health, including sleep. Sonia hopes to use her culinary abilities and wide knowledge to help others make informed nutritional choices that improve their quality of life.

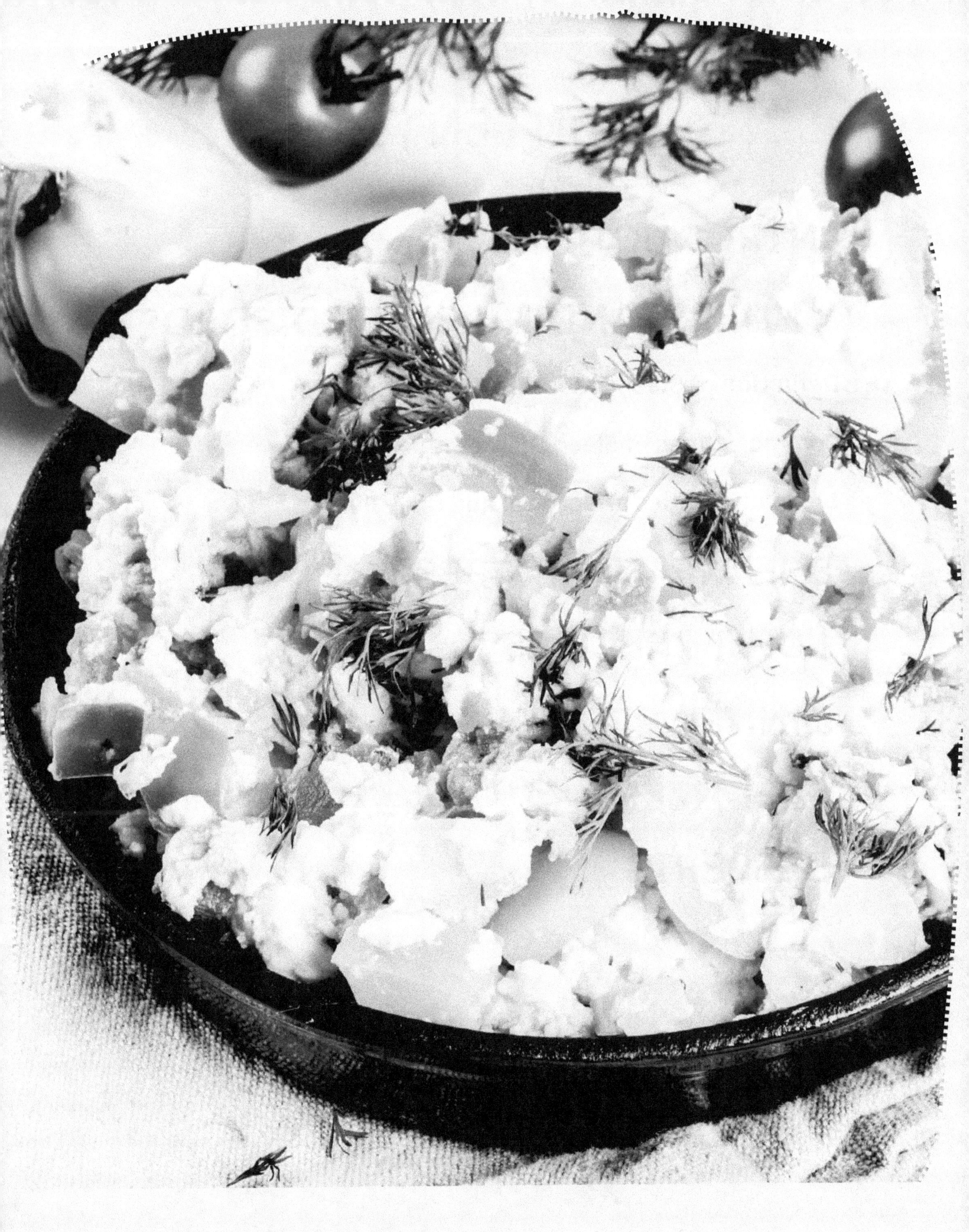

CONTENTS

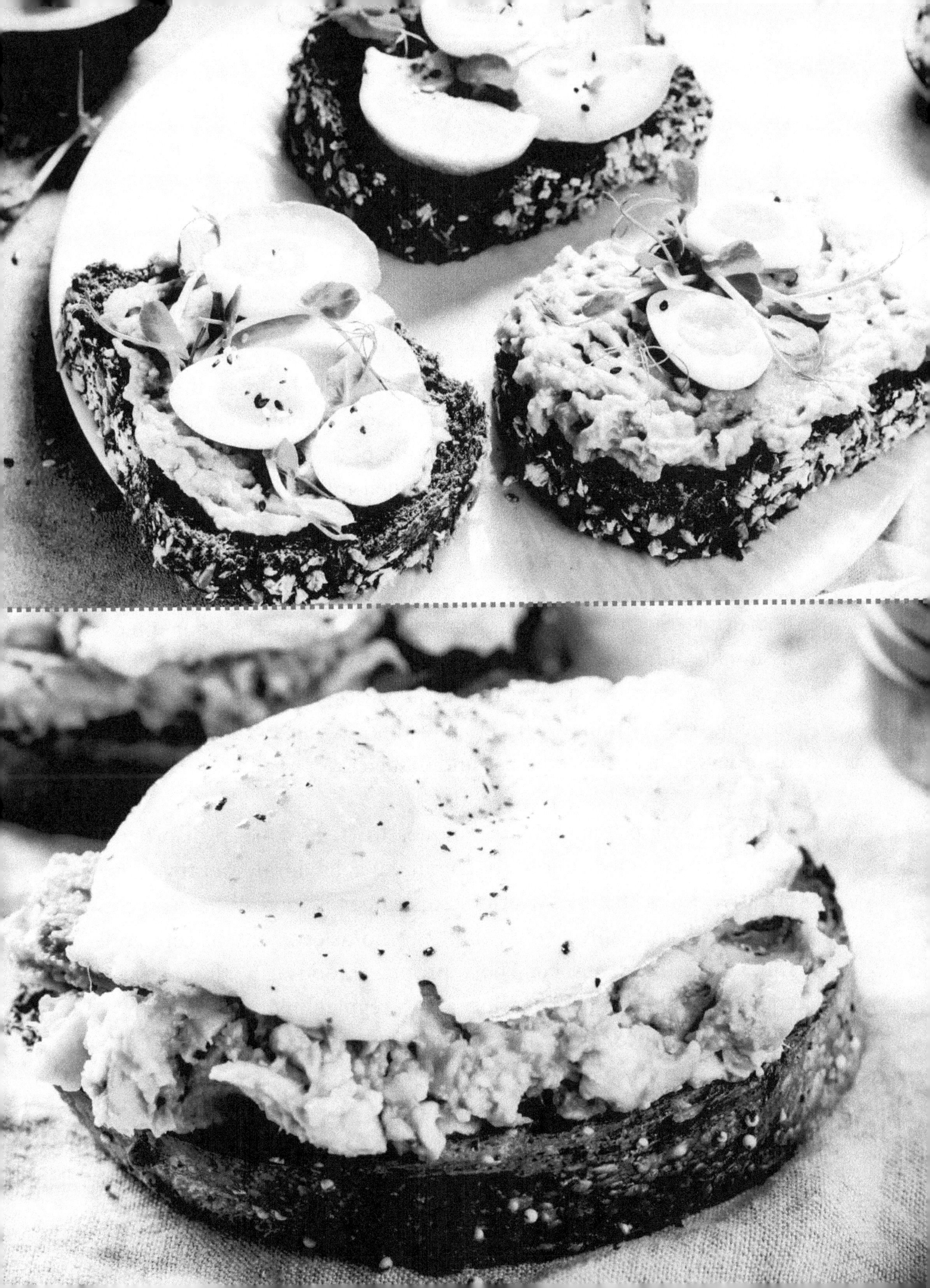

INTRODUCTION

Welcome to "Healthy Diet for Sleep Disorders: An In-depth Dietary Approach to Managing Sleep Disorders, Improving Sleep Quality, and Obtaining Better Health."If you've chosen this book, it's likely that you or someone you care about has difficulty sleeping. You are not alone. Millions of people throughout the world suffer from sleep disorders, which interrupt their lives and reduce their well-being.

Sleep is a critical component of total health, much like air, food, and drink. Sleep is when our bodies repair themselves, our minds assimilate information, and we prepare for the day ahead. When sleep is disrupted, it can trigger a series of health problems, ranging from chronic weariness and mood swings to more serious disorders such as heart disease and diabetes.

While there are numerous techniques to treating sleep disorders, ranging from medication to cognitive behavioral therapy, one effective and sometimes overlooked strategy is food. What you eat can significantly affect your ability to go asleep, stay asleep, and wake up feeling refreshed. The appropriate foods can stimulate the creation of sleep-enhancing hormones, regulate blood sugar levels, and supply critical nutrients for comfortable sleep.

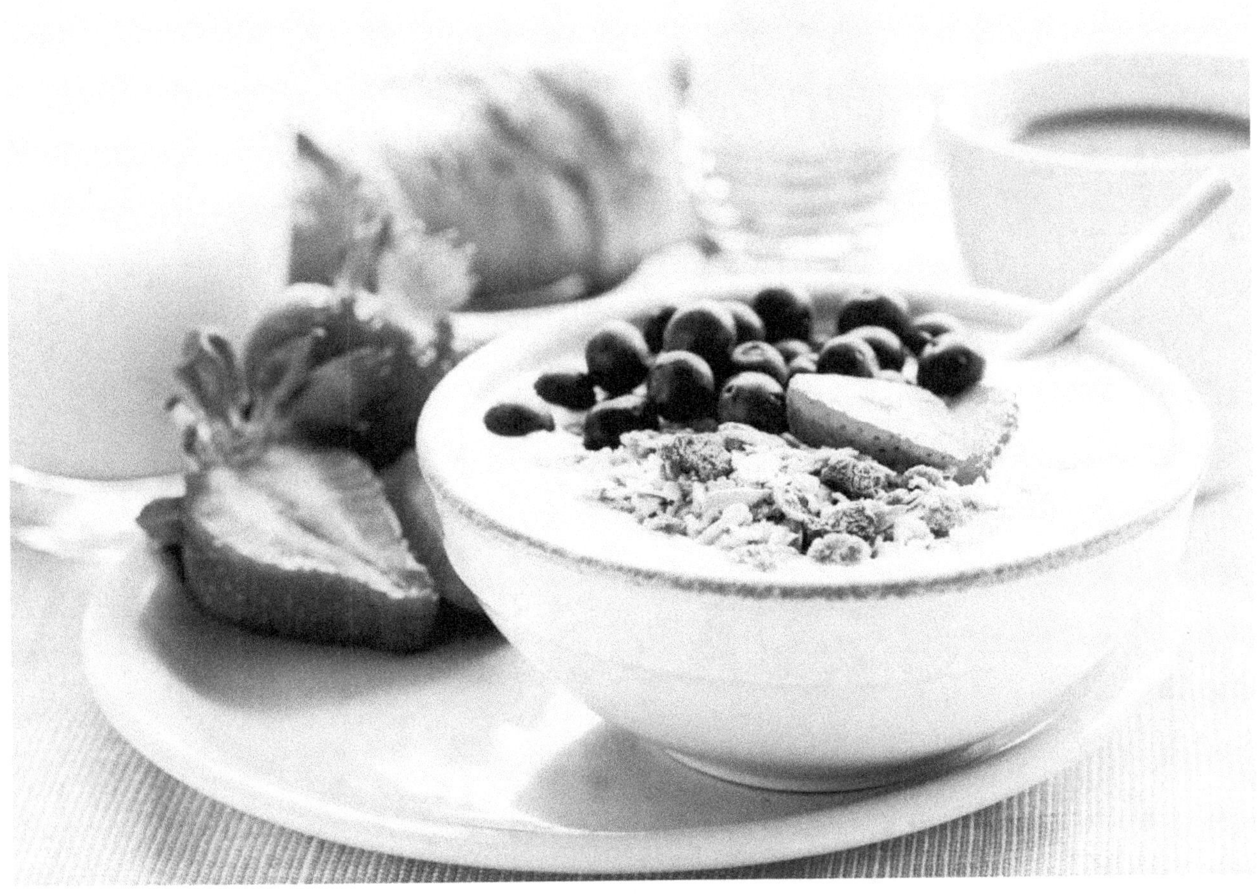

This book is intended to be a guide to understanding the complex relationship between nutrition and sleep. We will look at the science behind sleep problems, the nutrients that play an important role in sleep regulation, and practical dietary methods to help you sleep better. However, this is more than simply theory; it is also about action. You'll find a plethora of tasty, simple dishes designed to help you sleep better, ranging from full breakfasts to satisfying meals and everything in between.

I hope that this journey will help you take control of your sleep health through the power of diet. Let us take this journey together, to nights of deep, restorative sleep and days full of vitality and well-being

PART 1: UNDERSTANDING SLEEP DISORDERS

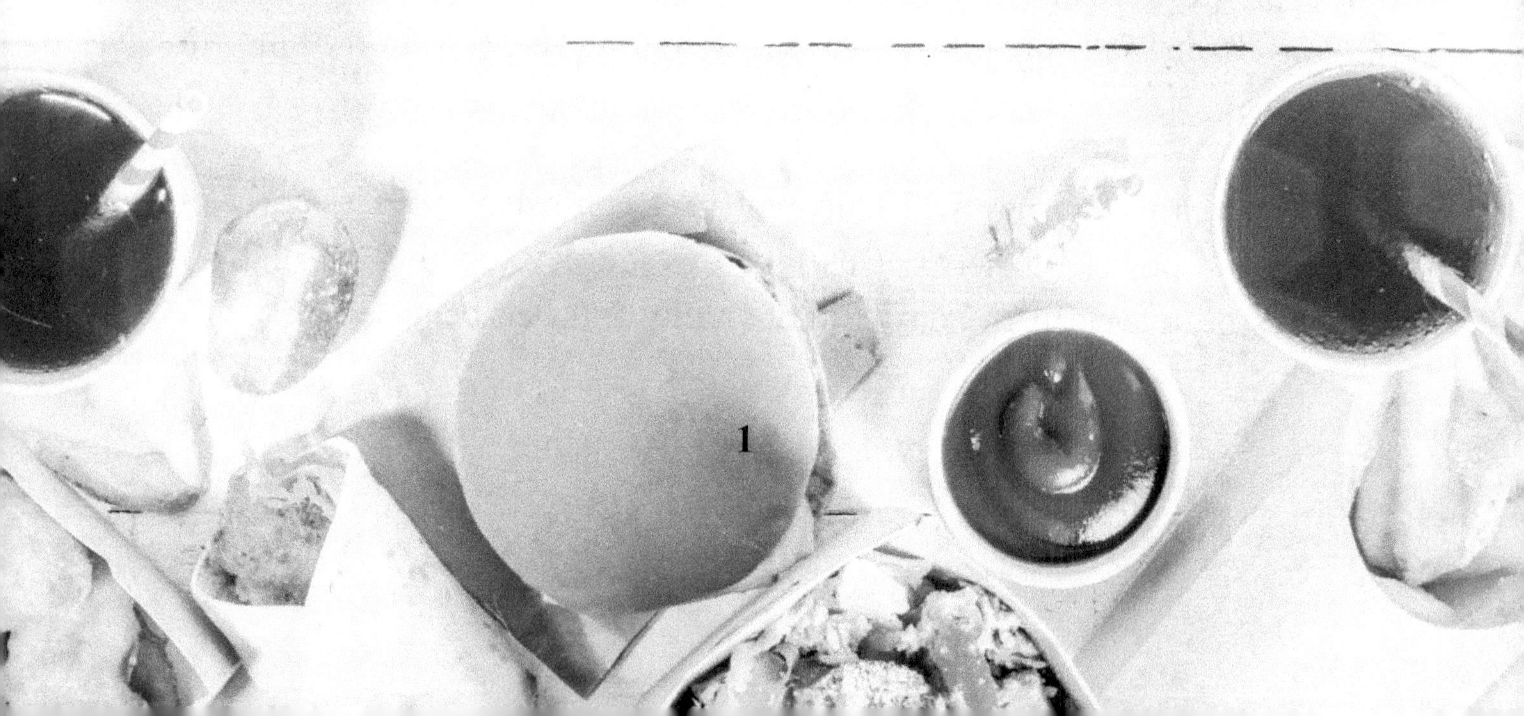

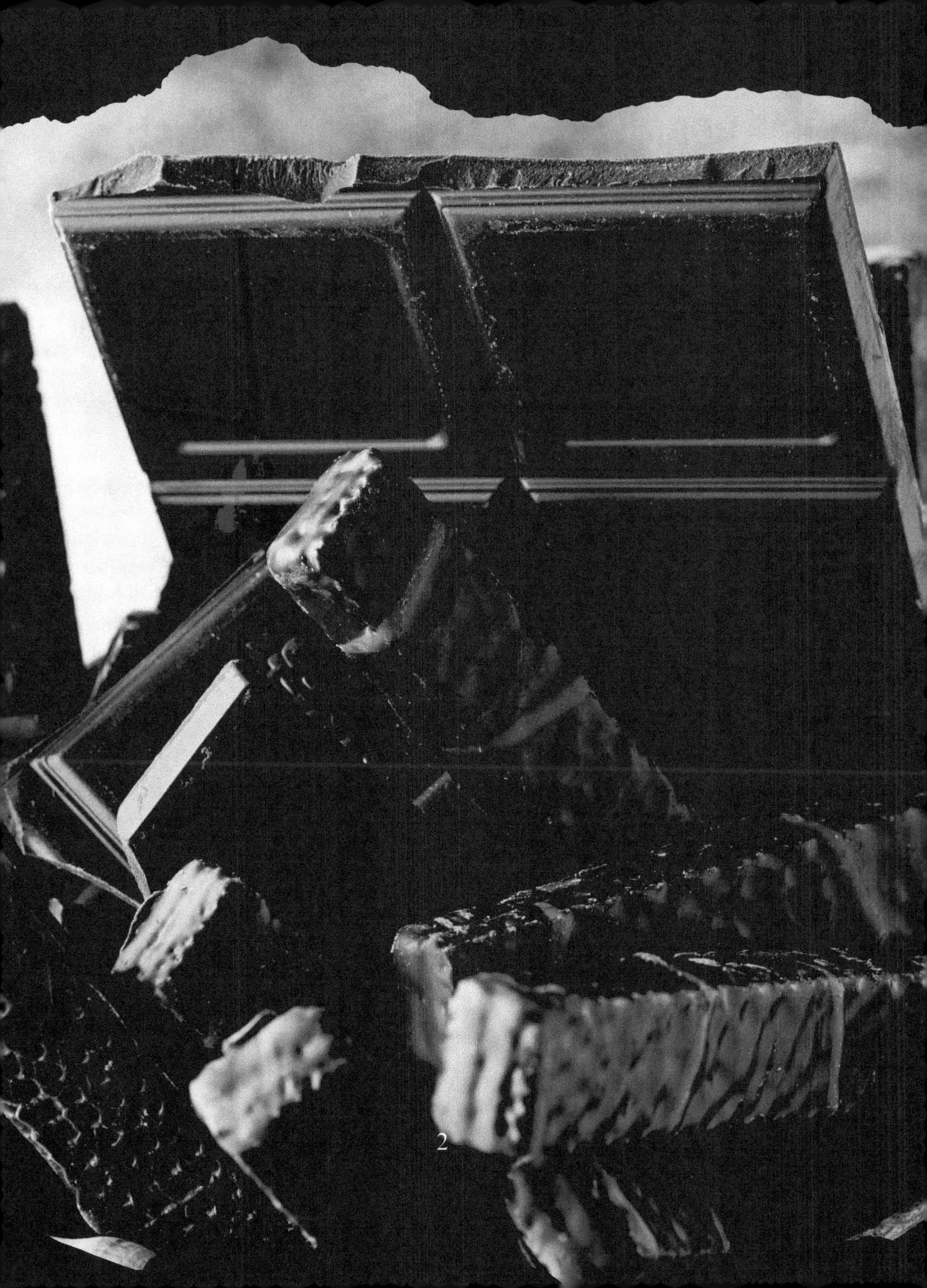

DEFINITION OF SLEEP DISORDER

Sleep disorders are a broad category of ailments that disrupt the quality, timing, and duration of sleep, resulting in daily distress and reduced functioning. These illnesses can affect people of all ages and are caused by a variety of variables such as lifestyle choices, physical ailments, psychological issues, and environmental effects. Understanding the many types of sleep disturbances is critical for developing effective treatment and management strategies.

Common Types of Sleep Disorders:

1. Insomnia: Insomnia is the most common sleep problem, defined as trouble getting asleep, staying asleep, or waking up too early and unable to fall back asleep. People with insomnia frequently report dissatisfaction with their sleep and may experience exhaustion, mood swings, and poor cognitive function during the day. Stress and anxiety, as well as poor sleeping habits and underlying health concerns, can all contribute to insomnia.

2. Sleep Apnea: Sleep apnea is a significant sleep disorder in which breathing stops and starts often during sleep. The most frequent variety is obstructive sleep apnea (OSA), which happens when the throat muscles relax and block the airway. Central sleep apnea is less prevalent and occurs when the brain fails to transmit correct signals to the muscles that govern breathing. Symptoms include loud snoring, gasping for air during sleeping, and excessive daytime tiredness.

3. Restless Legs Syndrome (RLS): RLS is a neurological illness defined by an involuntary impulse to move the legs, which is frequently accompanied by unpleasant sensations. These sensations usually occur in the evening or at night when you are resting, making it difficult to fall or stay asleep. Movement briefly alleviates the ache, but it might lead to disturbed sleep and afternoon weariness.

4. Narcolepsy: Narcolepsy is a persistent sleep condition characterized by excessive daytime sleepiness and unexpected sleep attacks. People suffering from narcolepsy may have cataplexy (sudden loss of muscle tone), sleep paralysis (temporary inability to move or talk while falling asleep or waking), and hallucinations. Narcolepsy is thought to be caused by the brain's failure to correctly regulate sleep and waking cycles.

5. Circadian Rhythm Sleep Disorders: These disorders are caused by a misalignment between an individual's internal biological clock and their surroundings. Examples include delayed sleep phase disorder (difficulty falling asleep and waking up at regular times), advanced sleep phase disorder (early sleep onset and wake times), and shift work disorder (sleep issues caused by irregular work hours).

6. Parasomnias: These are aberrant behaviors, movements, or experiences that occur while sleeping. Sleepwalking, night terrors, and REM sleep behavior disorder (acting out dreams) are examples of common parasomnias. These diseases can cause severe anguish and pose risks to both the sufferer and others.

The Impact of Sleep Disorders:

Sleep disturbances can have far-reaching effects for both physical and mental health. Chronic sleep deprivation and interrupted sleep can impair cognitive performance, decrease productivity, and raise the chance of an accident. Furthermore, untreated sleep difficulties have been related to a variety of health issues, including cardiovascular disease, diabetes, obesity, depression, and impaired immune function.

Diagnosis and treatments:

Sleep disorders are often diagnosed with a comprehensive evaluation that includes medical history, sleep diaries, physical examinations, and specialist testing such as polysomnography (sleep study) or actigraphy. Treatment options vary based on the disease and may include lifestyle changes, behavioral therapy, medical equipment (e.g., CPAP for sleep apnea), drugs, and nutritional changes.

Understanding sleep disorders and their consequences is the first step toward more effective management and better sleep quality. Individuals can dramatically improve their sleep and overall well-being by addressing the underlying causes and taking a comprehensive strategy that includes dietary changes.

COMMON SYMPTOMS AND CAUSES OF SLEEP DISORDERS

Sleep problems develop in a variety of ways, frequently presenting with a wide range of symptoms that can have a major impact on everyday living. Identifying these symptoms is critical for diagnosing a sleep issue and obtaining suitable therapy. Sleep disorders have a variety of reasons, including lifestyle choices, physical illnesses, psychological issues, and environmental effects.

Common Symptoms:

1. Difficulty Falling Asleep: One of the most common symptoms is difficulty starting sleep, which is frequently accompanied by feelings of restlessness and worry as bedtime approaches.

2. Frequent Nighttime Awakenings: People with sleep disorders may wake up several times during the night and struggle to fall back asleep.

3. Early Morning Awakenings: Waking up too early and being unable to fall back down is a common symptom, especially for insomnia.

4. Excessive Daytime Sleepiness: Consistent weariness and a strong desire to snooze during the day may suggest poor nightly sleep quality.

5. Loud snoring or gasping for air: These symptoms are frequently connected with sleep apnea, a condition in which breathing disruptions impair sleep.

6. Uncontrollable Leg Movements: In disorders such as Restless Legs Syndrome (RLS), people may have an insatiable desire to move their legs, particularly in the evening.

7. Abrupt Sleep Attacks: Narcolepsy is characterized by abrupt episodes of sleep that might occur at inappropriate times, such as during discussions or while driving.

8. Unusual Sleep Behaviors: Parasomnias include sleepwalking, night terrors, and acting out dreams (such as in REM sleep behavior disorder).

9. Difficulty Concentrating: Poor sleep quality frequently results in reduced cognitive processes, such as difficulty focusing, memory issues, and slower reaction times.

10. Mood Changes: Chronic sleep deprivation can result in irritation, anxiety, despair, and mood swings.

Common causes:

1. Stress and Anxiety: Being stressed and anxious might make it difficult to relax and sleep. Worries about job, money, relationships, or health might keep the mind awake at night.

2. Poor Sleep Habits: Irregular sleep cycles, excessive screen time before bedtime, and ingesting caffeine or large meals late in the evening can all disrupt sleep patterns.

3. Medical Conditions: Chronic conditions such as heart disease, diabetes, asthma, and gastroesophageal reflux disease (GERD) can disrupt sleep. Painful illnesses such as arthritis and fibromyalgia can sometimes cause sleep disruptions.

4. Sleep Apnea: Obstructive sleep apnea, caused by the relaxation of neck muscles resulting in obstructed airways, and central sleep apnea, caused by the brain's failure to regulate breathing, are both major causes of fragmented sleep.

5. Drugs: Some drugs used to treat hypertension, depression, asthma, and allergies can cause sleep disturbances.

6. Lifestyle Factors: Shift work, jet lag, and irregular sleep-wake routines can cause circadian rhythm disorders, in which the body's internal clock is out of sync with its surroundings.

7. Psychological difficulties: Sleep difficulties are frequently associated with depression, bipolar disorder, and other mental health issues. These disorders can affect sleep patterns and quality.

8. Neurological Disorders: Diseases including Parkinson's, Alzheimer's, and epilepsy can impair the brain's capacity to regulate sleep.

9. Substance Use: Alcohol, nicotine, and recreational substances can disrupt sleep architecture, resulting in poor sleep quality and overnight awakenings.

10. Environmental Factors: A noisy, uncomfortable, or disturbed sleeping environment can have a substantial impact on sleep quality. Room temperature, lighting, and bedding are all factors that can influence this.

Understanding Symptoms and Causes:

Recognizing the symptoms and underlying causes of sleep problems is critical for successful diagnosis and therapy. While some factors are beyond our control, many can be addressed with lifestyle modifications, medical interventions, and targeted medicines. Understanding the multidimensional nature of sleep problems allows people to take proactive actions toward better sleep hygiene, better health, and a higher quality of life.

SLEEP DIFFICULTIES AFFECT HEALTH AND DAILY LIVING.

Sleep disorders are often disregarded, yet they can have a significant impact on both physical health and daily living. The repercussions of insufficient or poor-quality sleep go beyond weariness, affecting several elements of well-being and general functioning. Understanding these consequences is critical for understanding the significance of managing sleep disorders and taking appropriate action to lessen their effects.

Physical health:

1. Cardiovascular Health: Chronic sleep loss, as well as sleep apnea, are associated with an increased risk of hypertension, heart disease, stroke, and irregular heartbeat. Poor sleep reduces the body's ability to control blood pressure and promotes inflammation, both of which are risk factors for cardiovascular disease.

2. Metabolic Health: A lack of sleep alters the balance of hormones that drive hunger and appetite, including ghrelin and leptin. This disruption can cause weight gain and obesity, which raises the risk of developing type 2 diabetes. Inadequate sleep also reduces insulin sensitivity, worsening metabolic problems.

3. Immune Function: Sleep is essential for a strong immune system. Chronic sleep deprivation impairs the immune system, making the body more vulnerable to diseases and reducing the efficiency of immunizations.

4. Mental Health: Sleep difficulties are strongly associated with mental health issues such as depression, anxiety, and bipolar disorder. Insomnia and other sleep disturbances can both cause and exacerbate these illnesses, resulting in a vicious cycle of poor sleep and deteriorating mental health.

5. Pain Perception: Insufficient sleep can lower the pain threshold and increase sensitivity to pain, increasing chronic pain illnesses such as arthritis and fibromyalgia. In contrast, pain can disrupt sleep, resulting in a vicious cycle of discomfort and insomnia.

Cognitive Function and Performance:

1. Attention and focus: Sleep disorders decrease cognitive functioning like attention, focus, and problem-solving ability. This can have an impact on job performance, academic accomplishment, and the capacity to complete daily chores efficiently.

2. Memory: Sleep is necessary for memory consolidation, which is the process by which short-term memories are converted into long-term ones. Disrupted sleep disrupts this process, causing amnesia and trouble remembering new information.

3. Decision-Making: Sleep deprivation affects the prefrontal cortex, the brain region in charge of decision-making, impulse control, and judgment. This can result in poor decision-making and risk-taking behaviors.

4. Reaction Time: Sleep deprivation causes slower reaction times, which is especially harmful for occupations that require quick responses, such as driving. Drunken driving is a major cause of traffic accidents and fatalities.

Emotional and Social Wellbeing:

1. Mood Stability: Inadequate sleep can cause irritation, mood swings, and increased emotional reactivity. This can affect relationships with family, friends, and coworkers, resulting in social isolation and conflict.

2. Stress Management: Getting enough sleep is vital for dealing with stress. Sleep difficulties can diminish resilience to stress, making it more difficult to manage daily challenges and raising the risk of burnout.

3. Quality of Life: Chronic sleep disorders can have a major impact on overall quality of life, limiting enjoyment of everyday activities and decreasing life satisfaction.

Daily Functioning:

1. Productivity: Sleep disorders limit productivity at work or school, resulting in missed deadlines, worse quality work, and higher absenteeism. The economic cost of missed production due to sleep disorders is significant.

2. Energy Levels: Persistent weariness and low energy levels might make it difficult to engage in physical activities and sustain an active lifestyle, contributing to sedentary behavior and related health issues.

3. Safety: Sleep difficulties raise the risk of accidents and injuries, both at home and at work. Sleep deprivation can cause a loss of alertness and coordination, which can lead to falls, machinery mishandling, and other mishaps.

Recognizing the widespread effects of sleep problems is the first step toward effective management and prevention. Addressing sleep disorders with lifestyle modifications, medicinal therapies, and dietary interventions can greatly improve sleep quality, overall health, and everyday functioning. Individuals who prioritize sleep health can get the benefits of deep, restorative sleep and enjoy more productive, meaningful lives.

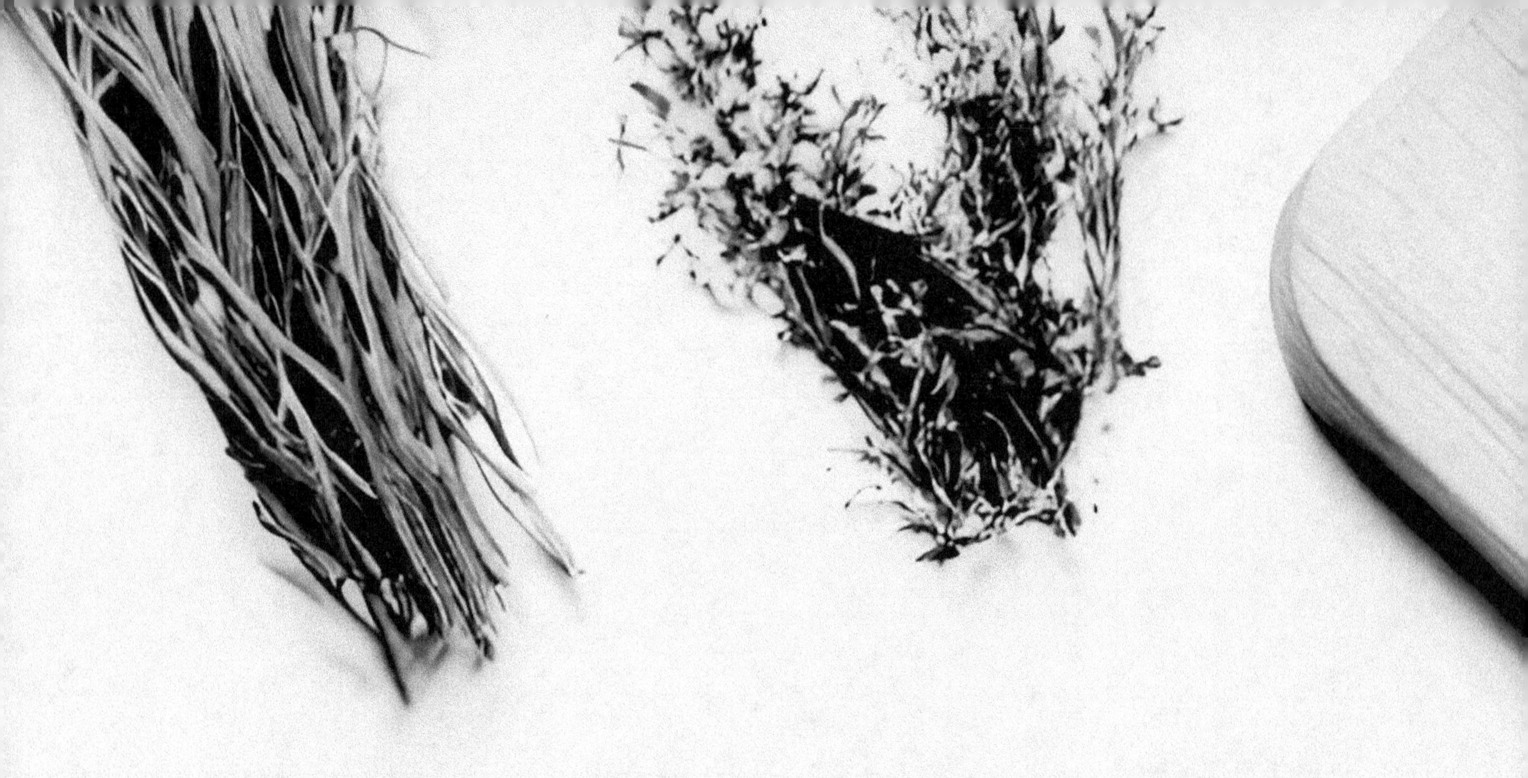

BREAKFAST RECIPES

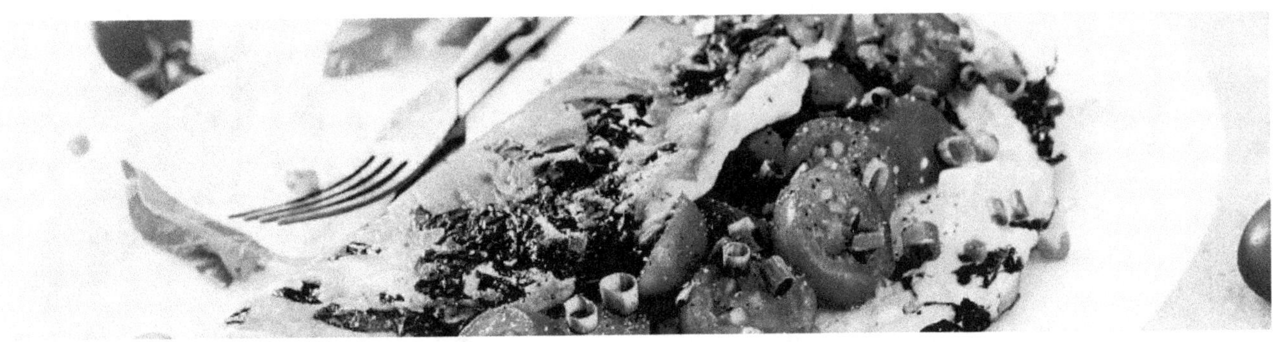

Scrambled eggs with spinach and feta

CALORIES: 250   **FAT: 19G**   **PROTEIN: 16G**   **CARB: 4G**

SERVINGS: 2   **COOK TIME: 5 MINS**   **TOTAL TIME: 5 MINS**

INGREDIENTS

4 ounces of fresh spinach.

Four big eggs.

1 tablespoon butter.

1 ounce. feta.

1 pinch of crushed red

pepper.

1 pinch of freshly cracked

black pepper.

1 pinch of salt.

DIRECTIONS

1. Roughly chop the spinach into 1-inch pieces. This step is optional and can be avoided to speed up breakfast, but I prefer smaller pieces that do not become stringy, as full spinach leaves can.
2. Crack the eggs into a large mixing bowl, season with salt, and whisk until combined.
3. Melt the butter in a large skillet over medium heat. Sauté the chopped spinach until it softens (2-3 minutes).
4. Push the sautéed spinach to the skillet's edges and pour the eggs in the center.
5. Gently fold the eggs until the bottom layer is about 75% solid. Fold the eggs into the sautéed spinach and turn off the heat. The remaining heat in the pan will cook the eggs without overcooking or drying them out.
6. Serve the eggs with crumbled feta, a sprinkle of freshly cracked pepper, and a pinch of crushed red pepper.

16

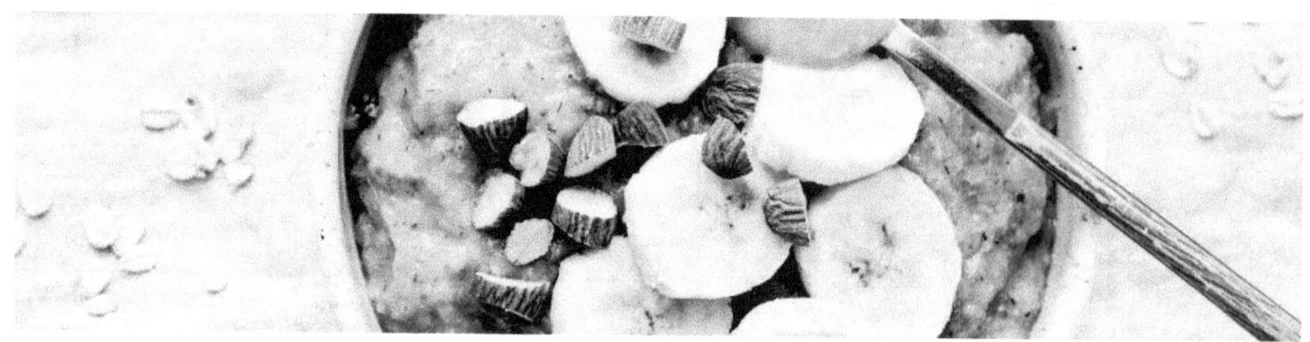

Oatmeal with almond butter and banana

CALORIES: 592   **FAT: 23G**   **PROTEIN: 9G**   **CARB: 87G**

SERVINGS: 1   **PREP TIME: 5 MINS**   **COOK TIME: 5 MINS**

INGREDIENTS

Oatmeal
1/2 cup old-fashioned oatmeal
Add 1 cup water and a pinch of salt.
1/2 teaspoon of vanilla extract.
1/4 teaspoon cinnamon.
Toppings
One banana, sliced
2 tablespoons maple syrup
1 tablespoon almond butter.
2 tablespoons granola.
1 tablespoon crushed walnuts, chia seeds, and a pinch of cinnamon.

DIRECTIONS

1. Bring a pot of 1 cup water to a boil on the stovetop. Mix in 1/2 cup oats, a touch of salt, vanilla, and cinnamon. Let simmer for 5 minutes, stirring occasionally.
2. Serve in a bowl and garnish with banana slices, granola, nuts and seeds, and maple syrup.

> **Tip:** Toppings can include peanut butter or cashew butter, nuts, your favorite granola, and any additional fruit you choose.

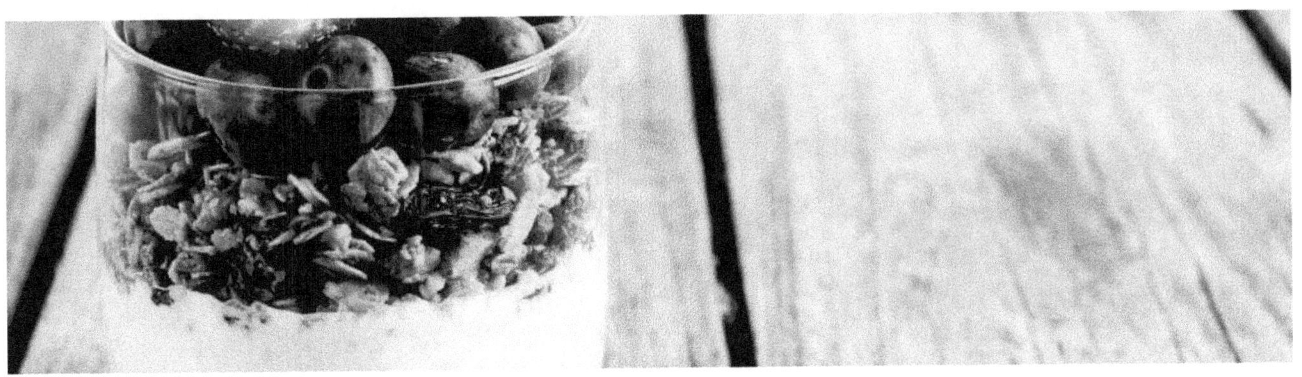

Greek yogurt with berries and chia seeds

CALORIES: 415   **FAT: 19G**   **PROTEIN: 23G**   **CARB: 38G**

SERVINGS: 1   **PREP TIME: 5 MINS**   **TOTAL TIME: 5 MINS**

INGREDIENTS

1/2 cup yogurt of your choosing.
1/2 cup milk of choice.
1/2 cup frozen wild blueberries.
1–3 tablespoons raw honey or maple syrup (optional)
½ teaspoon vanilla extract.
Tiny pinch of fine sea salt.
3 tablespoons chia seeds.

TOPPING IDEAS

Granola with sliced bananas
Nut Butter
Berries Nuts or seeds (such as walnuts, hemp, and sunflower seeds).

DIRECTIONS

1. In an upright blender, combine the yogurt, milk, blueberries, sweetener (if desired), vanilla, and salt. Blend until smooth. Pour into a jar and add the chia seeds. Whisk until combined.
2. If possible, stir every couple of hours until the mixture has thickened to your desire. I just froze mine overnight and stirred it well in the morning!
3. Add your favorite toppings and devour it!

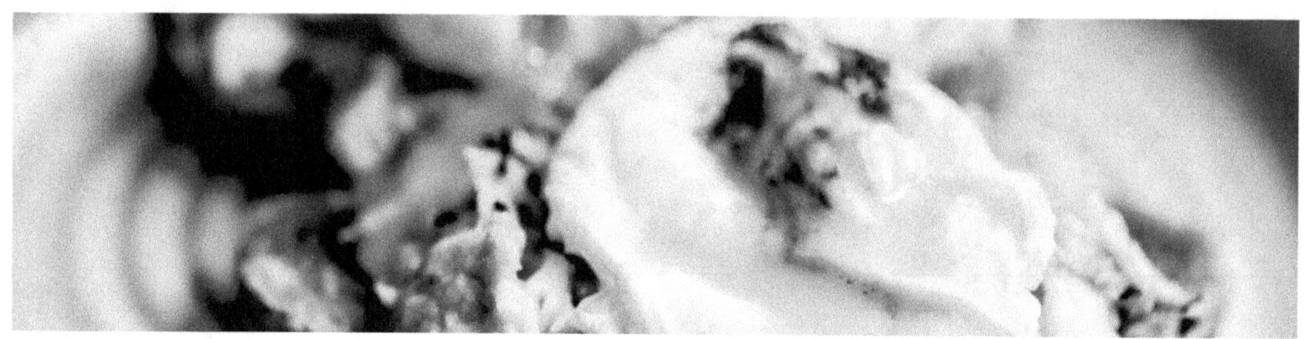

Poached egg and avocado toast

CALORIES: 271   **FAT: 20.4G**   **PROTEIN: 23.3G**   **CARB: 30.1G**

SERVINGS: 1   **PREP TIME: 5 MINS**   **TOTAL TIME: 5 MINS**

INGREDIENTS

2 eggs

2 pieces of whole grain bread.

1/3 avocado (I normally cut it in half but don't use the whole thing. Okay, maybe I do.

2 tablespoons shredded Parmesan cheese

Salt and pepper for the topping.

Top with fresh herbs (parsley, thyme, or basil).

Quartered heirloom tomatoes for serving.

DIRECTIONS

1. Bring a kettle of water to a boil (enough to cover the eggs when they are placed in the bottom). Drop the metal rims (outer rim only) of two mason jar lids into the pot, ensuring they are flat on the bottom. When the water is boiling, turn off the heat and carefully crack the eggs into each rim. Cover the saucepan and cook for 5 minutes (4 for ultra soft, 4:30 for soft, and 5 or more for semi-soft yolks).
2. While the eggs are cooking, toast the bread and spread the avocado on each slice. When the eggs are finished, use a spatula to remove them out of the water. Gently remove the rims of the eggs (I do this right on the spatula, over the water) and serve the poached eggs on top of the toast. Sprinkle with Parmesan cheese, salt, pepper, and fresh herbs; serve with freshly quartered heirloom tomatoes.

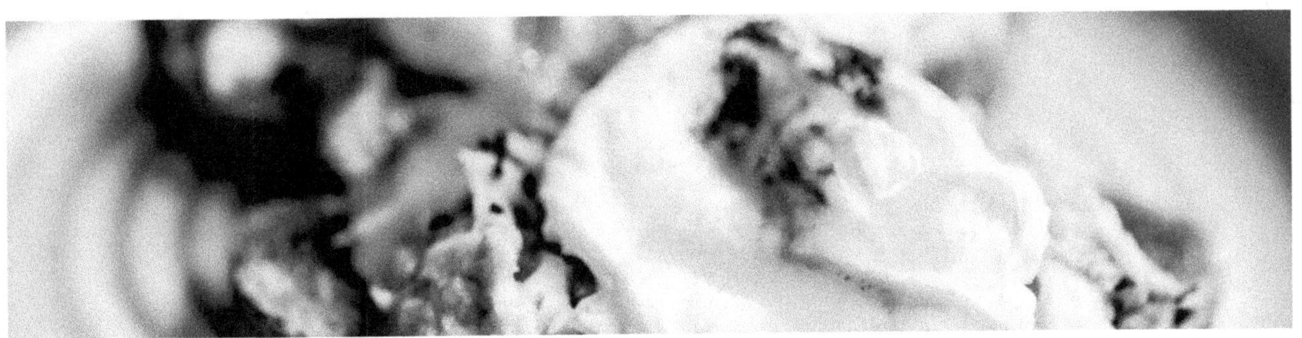

Tip: Toppings can include peanut
butter or cashew butter, nuts, your
favorite granola, and any additional
fruit you choose.

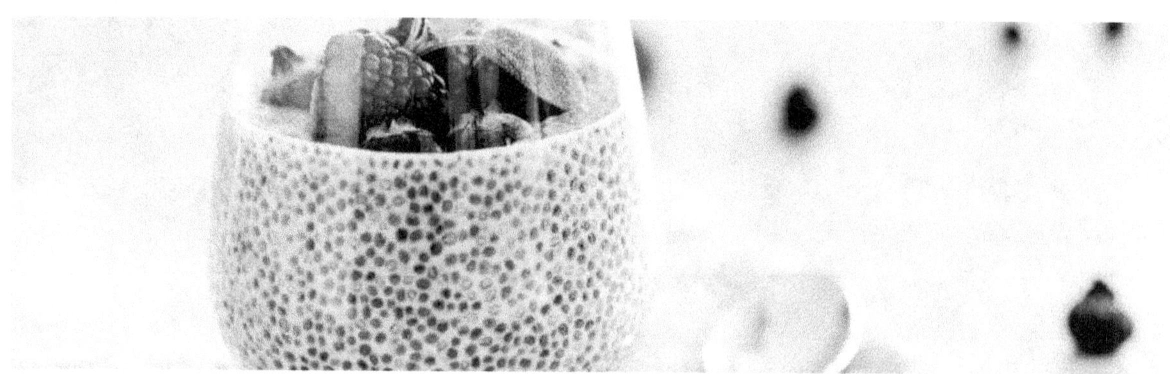

Chia Seed Pudding with Fresh Fruit

CALORIES: 216   **FAT: 17G**   **PROTEIN: 3G**   **CARB: 17G**

SERVINGS: 3   **PREP TIME: 10 MINS**   **TOTAL TIME: 10 MINS**

INGREDIENTS

Use 3/4 cup full-fat coconut milk. 1/2 tablespoons pure maple syrup
1/2 teaspoon vanilla extract
Add 3 tablespoons of chia seeds and diced fresh fruit, such as blueberries, strawberries, and blackberries.

DIRECTIONS

1. In a large mixing basin, whisk together the coconut milk, maple syrup, and vanilla extract until thoroughly combined.
2. Whisk in the chia seeds.
3. Pour the mixture into two or three serving bowls or glasses, depending on their size. Allow it to settle for approximately 30 minutes at room temperature.
4. Refrigerate for at least 3 hours, preferably overnight.
5. Remove the dishes from the refrigerator about 15 minutes before serving. Top with fresh fruit and serve!

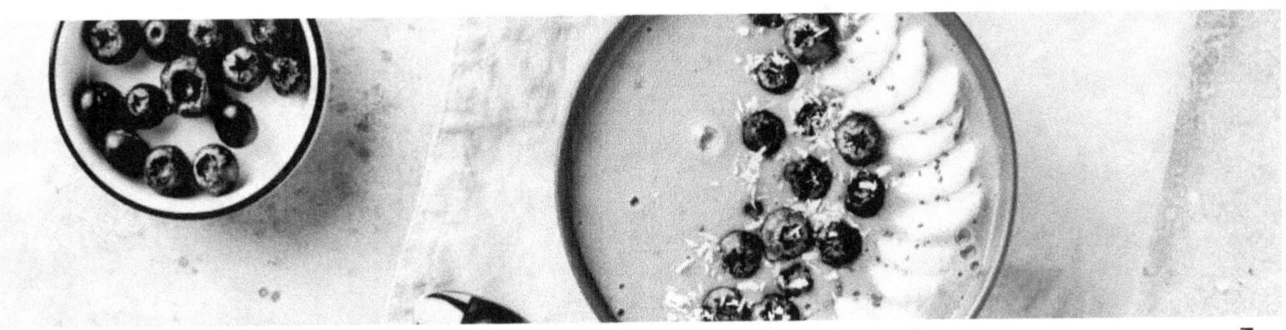

Smoothie bowl with spinach, banana, and protein-rich ingredients

CALORIES: 288 **FAT: 12G** **PROTEIN: 6G** **CARB: 46G**

SERVINGS: 1 **PREP TIME: 8 MINS** **COOK TIME: 2 MINS**

INGREDIENTS

For the smoothie bowl:

1/2 cup unsweetened vanilla almond milk
or any other milk of your choosing.
For this recipe, use 1 cup of fresh spinach
and 1/2 cup of frozen banana pieces.
1 cup frozen mixed berries.
1 tablespoon almond butter. Peanut
butter, or your favorite nut butter.
Optional: ½-1 scoop of protein powder.
Optional: ½-1 tablespoon honey or pure
maple syrup.
A powerful blender, such as a Vitamix

For toppings (choose all or a few)

Fresh banana slices.
Fresh berries, including blueberries,
raspberries, and/or sliced strawberries.
2 tbsp granola.
2 teaspoons of chia seeds.
Drizzle almond or peanut butter.

DIRECTIONS

1. In a high-powered blender, combine the smoothie bowl components in the following order: almond milk, spinach, banana, berries, almond butter, and protein powder. Blend until smooth. The smoothie will be really thick. Stop to scrape down the blender as needed, and add a little more almond milk if it becomes entirely stuck. Taste the smoothie, and if you want it sweeter, add honey or pure maple syrup until you reach your desired sweetness.

2. Scrape into a serving bowl. Add any preferred toppings. Enjoy right away.

22

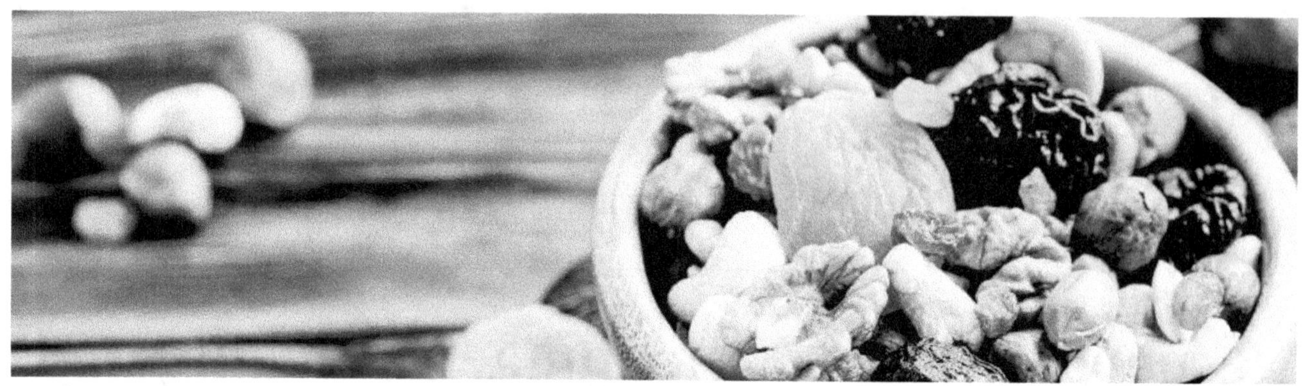

Quinoa breakfast bowl with mixed nuts and dried fruit.

SERVINGS: 4   **PREP TIME: 15 MINS**   **COOK TIME: 10 MINS**

INGREDIENTS

2 cups of cooked quinoa.
1 cup of unsweetened almond milk.
2 tablespoons of chopped nuts, like almonds, pecans, or walnuts.
2 tablespoons seeds of pumpkin, sunflower, or hemp
2 tablespoons of dried fruit, such as raisins, cranberries, or blueberries.
1 teaspoon ground cinnamon.
½ teaspoon ground ginger.
2 tablespoons genuine maple syrup
1/2 cup fresh fruit, such as blueberries or strawberries.

DIRECTIONS

1. Cook the quinoa, almond milk, almonds, seeds, dried fruit, cinnamon, and ginger in a medium-sized pot over medium heat. Cook for around 10 minutes, or until the grains soften and the fruit plumps up.
2. Top with maple syrup and the freshest berries. Serve hot.

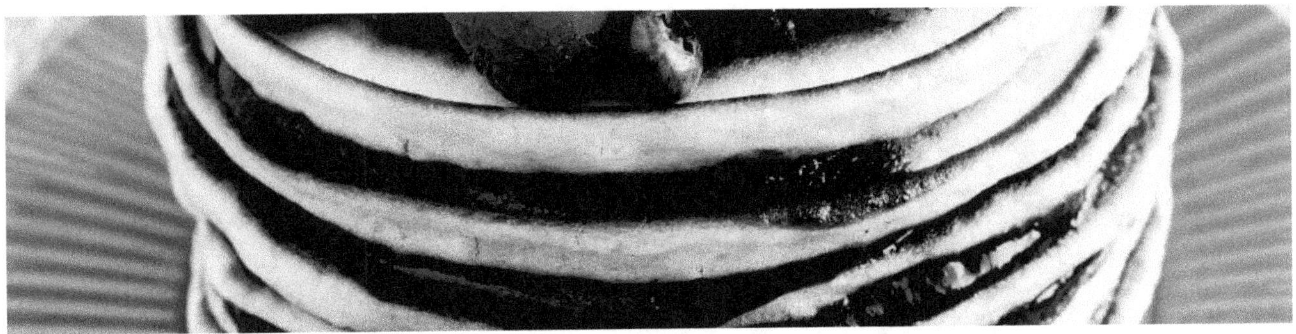

Whole Wheat Pancakes with Blueberry Compote

CALORIES: 474.3   **FAT: 19G**   **PROTEIN: 13.2G**   **CARB: 66G**

SERVINGS: 5   **COOK TIME: 15 MINS**   **TOTAL TIME: 15 MINS**

INGREDIENTS

PANCAKES

¾ cup all-purpose white flour
½ cup whole wheat flour
1 ½ tablespoons baking powder
½ teaspoon baking soda
1 teaspoon ground cinnamon.
1 teaspoon of coarse salt.
2 teaspoons sugar.
2 teaspoons of wheat germ.
1 1/2 cups soy milk (optional:
low-fat buttermilk or 2% milk)
Two eggs, lightly beaten
1/4 cup canola oil.

BLUEBERRY COMPOTE.

2 cups blueberries (fresh or
frozen; approximately 1 pint)
4 teaspoons of lemon juice.
1/8 teaspoon coarse salt.
1/4 cup sugar

DIRECTIONS

1. To create the pancakes, mix together the flours, wheat germ, sugar, baking powder, baking soda, cinnamon, and salt in a bowl. Mix in the milk, oil, and eggs. Allow the batter to rest for 10 minutes (if it thickens, add 1 tablespoon water).

2. To create the compote, combine blueberries, lemon juice, and salt in a skillet and cook over medium heat until the berries burst, about 4 to 5 minutes. Stir in the sugar. Simmer, stirring frequently, until thick enough to coat the back of a spoon, about 6 to 8 minutes. Transfer to a bowl.

3. To make the pancakes, coat a nonstick skillet with cooking spray and heat over medium heat. For each pancake, spoon in 1/4 cup batter. Cook until bubbles form. Flip and cook for about 2 minutes, or until golden brown. Serve immediately, or keep warm in a preheated oven. Drizzle compote over a plate of pancakes.

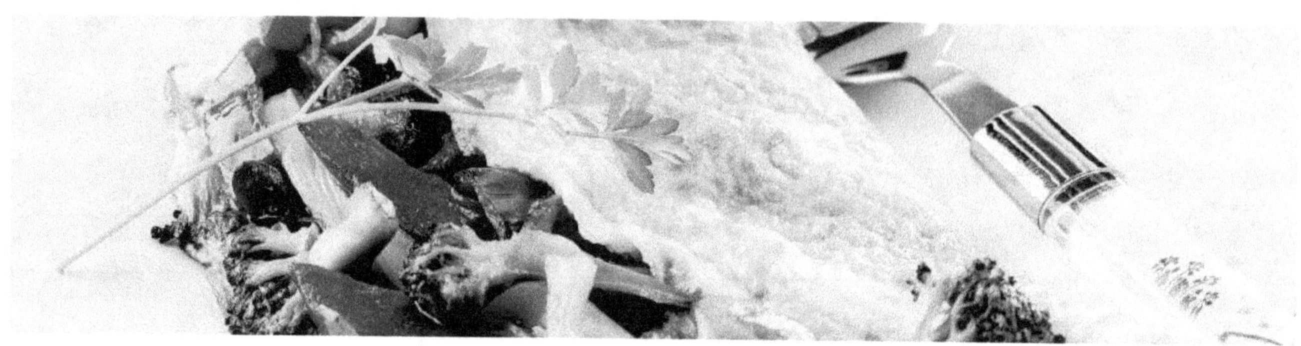

Vegetarian Omelet

CALORIES: 386   **FAT: 30G**   **PROTEIN: 22G**   **CARB: 9G**

SERVINGS: 2   **PREP TIME: 10 MINS**   **COOK TIME: 10 MINS**

INGREDIENTS

2 Tbsp butter, divided

1 small onion, chopped.

One green bell pepper, chopped

¾ teaspoon salt, divided.

Four big eggs.

Two teaspoons of milk

⅛ teaspoon fresh ground black pepper

2 ounces of shredded Swiss cheese.

DIRECTIONS

1. Melt 1 tablespoon butter in a medium skillet over medium heat. Cook and toss the onion and bell pepper in butter until just soft, about 4 to 5 minutes. Place vegetables in a bowl, season with 1/4 teaspoon salt, and put aside.
2. In a separate bowl, whisk together eggs, milk, the remaining 1/2 teaspoon salt, and pepper.
3. Melt the remaining 1 tablespoon butter in the skillet over medium heat, swirling to cover the bottom with butter. When the butter is bubbling, add the egg mixture and cook for about 1 minute, or until the bottom of the eggs begin to set. Gently raise the omelet's edges with a spatula to allow any raw egg to drip onto the griddle. Continue cooking for another 1 to 2 minutes, or until the middle of the omelet seems dry.
4. Sprinkle cheese over the omelet, then spread the veggie mixture over half of it. Use a spatula to carefully fold the omelet over the vegetables. Cook for approximately 1 minute, or until the cheese melts to the desired consistency. Slide the omelet onto a plate. Cut into halves and serve

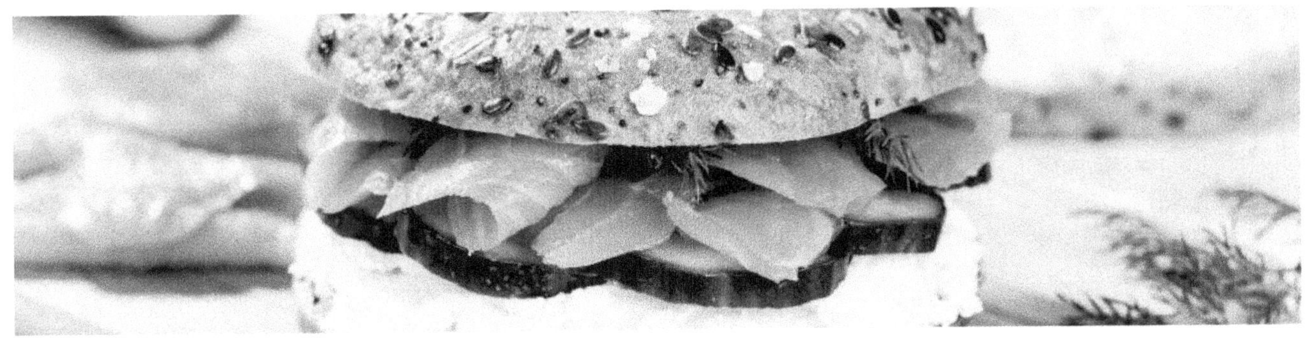

Smoked Salmon with Cream Cheese Bagel

CALORIES: 577   **FAT: 24G**   **PROTEIN: 26G**   **CARB: 64G**

SERVINGS: 2   **PREP TIME: 10 MINS**   **TOTAL TIME: 10 MINS**

INGREDIENTS

2 halved bagels

4 ounces thinly sliced smoked salmon

4 ounces cream cheese

2 tablespoons lemon juice

1 tablespoon fresh dill (plus more for serving)Season with salt and pepper to taste.

1-2 Persian cucumbers, red onion slices, and capers to taste.

DIRECTIONS

1. In a small bowl, mix together the cream cheese, lemon juice, fresh dill, and salt and pepper to taste.

2. Toast the bagels, then spread the cream cheese mixture on both sides of each. Spread the cucumbers, smoked salmon, capers, and red onions on the bottoms of the toasted bagels. Top with the top of the bagels.

Tip: Make ahead: This is best served immediately, but it will keep in the fridge for 24 hours if firmly covered.

Pineapple Cottage Cheese Bowl.

CALORIES: 244   **FAT: 12G**   **PROTEIN: 17G**   **CARB: 18G**

SERVINGS: 1   **PREP TIME: 10 MINS**   **TOTAL TIME: 10 MINS**

INGREDIENTS

1/2 cup low-fat cottage cheese.

¼ cup chopped fresh pineapple

1 tablespoon of unsweetened toasted coconut.

1 tablespoon of finely chopped macadamia nuts.

One tablespoon of granola

DIRECTIONS

1. Place cottage cheese in a small bowl. Arrange the pineapple, coconut, macadamia nuts, and granola over top. Serve immediately.

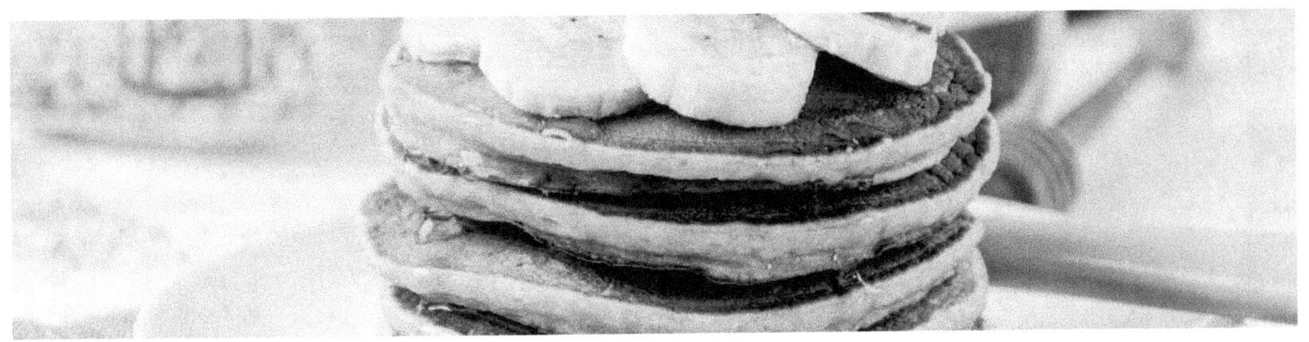

Banana Pancakes with Greek Yogurt

CALORIES: 81　　　**FAT: 1G**　　　**PROTEIN: 4G**　　　**CARB: 13G**

SERVINGS: 12　　　**COOK TIME: 10 MINS**　　　**TOTAL TIME: 20 MINS**

INGREDIENTS

12 oz vanilla Greek yogurt,
2 eggs, 1 cup white whole wheat
flour
2 teaspoons baking soda
1/2 cup milk (unsweetened
almond milk)
1 medium mashed banana

DIRECTIONS

1. In a medium-sized bowl, combine the Greek yogurt and the eggs. Whisk until combined.
2. In a separate basin, combine the flour and baking soda.
3. Pour the yogurt mixture over the dry ingredients and mix thoroughly. Add the milk and mashed banana, and stir thoroughly.
4. Heat a big skillet on the stove over medium heat, or set an electric griddle to 350 degrees. Melt a little butter in the skillet or on the griddle, then scoop the batter on top in the desired sizes. (I use a heaping 1/4 cup scoop and spread them out somewhat.)
5. Once the tops begin to bubble, flip and heat until both sides are thoroughly done. Serve alongside maple syrup, jam, almond butter, or fresh fruit.

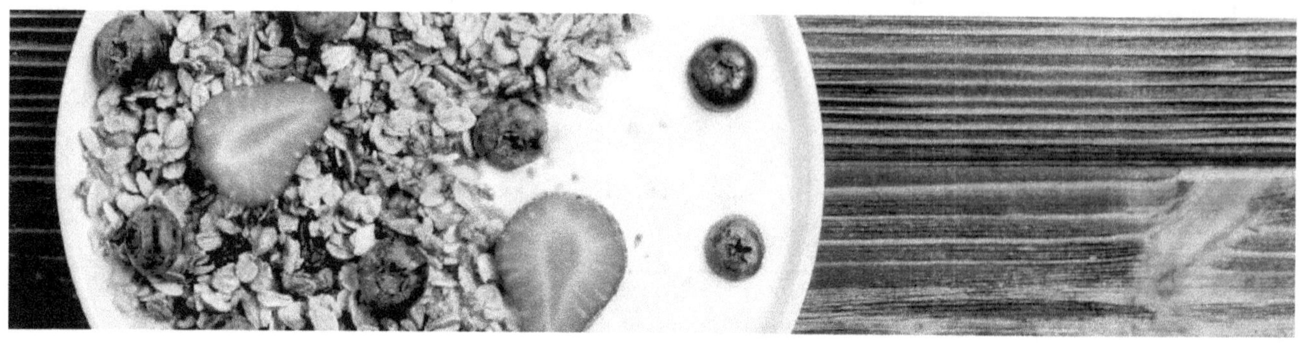

Acai Bowl With Granola And Mixed Berries

CALORIES: 281   **FAT: 7G**   **PROTEIN: 4G**   **CARB: 54G**

SERVINGS: 1   **PREP TIME: 5 MINS**   **TOTAL TIME: 5 MINS**

INGREDIENTS

Acai Bowl
1/2 cup coconut water.
One tiny frozen banana.
1 cup frozen strawberries
1 handful of fresh spinach.
1 tablespoon of acai powder.
½ teaspoon of maca powder.

TOPPINGS

¼ cup granola
½ small banana, thinly sliced
8–10 fresh berries
Fresh mint.
1 tablespoon of unsweetened
shredded coconut.
1 tablespoon of hemp hearts.

DIRECTIONS

1. Combine all of the smoothie ingredients in a blender or food processor and pulse until totally smooth. The smoothie should be thick, like soft-serve ice cream.
2. Pour into a bowl and top with your desired toppings. Serve immediately.

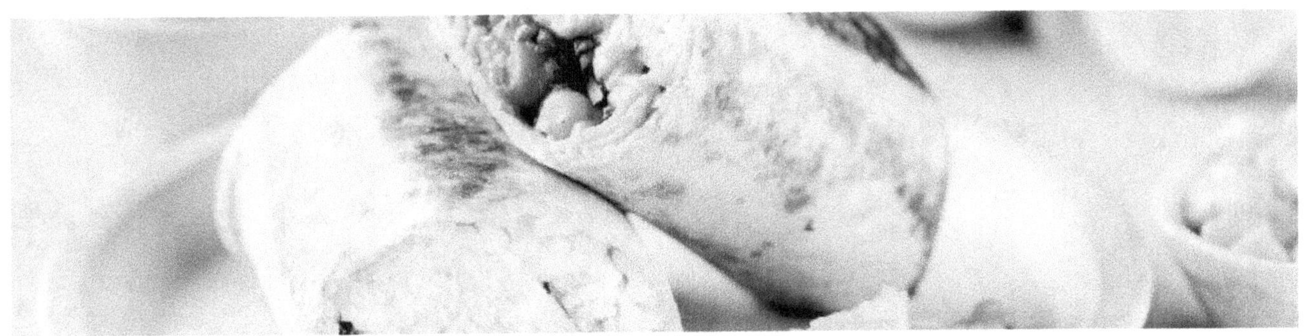

Egg and Spinach Breakfast Wrap

CALORIES: 304 **FAT: 11G** **PROTEIN: 23G** **CARB: 25G**

SERVINGS: 1 **PREP TIME: 10 MINS** **TOTAL TIME: 15 MINS**

INGREDIENTS

Use one whole grain or grain-free tortilla, such as Seite's burrito size tortillas.

Use 1-2 tablespoons of any flavor hummus.

1 egg, ¼ cup egg whites, ⅛ cup chopped onion

2 sliced button mushrooms, 2 cups baby spinach

1 tablespoon crumbled feta, 1 tablespoon chopped sun-dried tomatoes, sea salt and pepper to taste, and hot sauce for topping.

DIRECTIONS

1. Spray a skillet with cooking spray and sauté the onion and mushrooms for 3-4 minutes, until aromatic. Add the spinach and sauté for a few more minutes, or until wilted.
2. Cook the egg and egg whites in the pan with the vegetables for about 2 minutes, or until the eggs are fully cooked. While cooking, season with sea salt and ground pepper.
3. Warm the tortilla and apply a layer of hummus. Place the egg scramble in the center of the tortilla, then top with sun-dried tomatoes and feta. Sprinkle with additional salt and pepper, as well as any hot sauce you're using.
4. Wrap the tortilla up and serve!

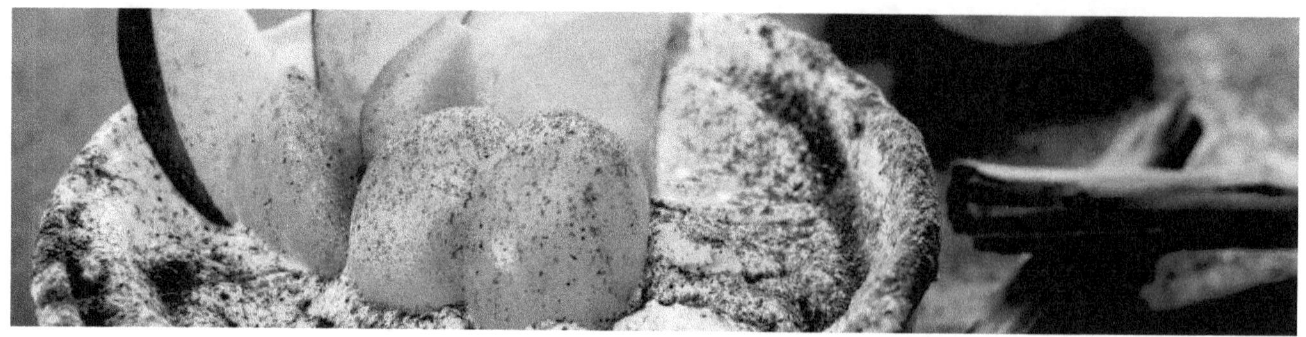

Sweet Potato, Greek Yogurt, and Cinnamon

CALORIES: 240   **FAT: 10G**   **PROTEIN: 10G**   **CARB: 0.5G**

SERVINGS: 4   **PREP TIME: 15 MINS**   **COOK TIME: 10 MINS**

INGREDIENTS

Four small to medium-sized
sweet potatoes baked
5.3 ounce Greek yogurt, plain or
vanilla.
2 teaspoons of honey.
½ teaspoon cinnamon
¼ teaspoon vanilla
Toast 1/2 cup of chopped pecans.

DIRECTIONS

1. In a small bowl, combine the yogurt, honey, cinnamon, and vanilla.
2. Cut sweet potatoes open and distribute the yogurt mixture between them.
3. Mix into the potato until fully combined.
4. Divide pecans among potatoes and serve hot

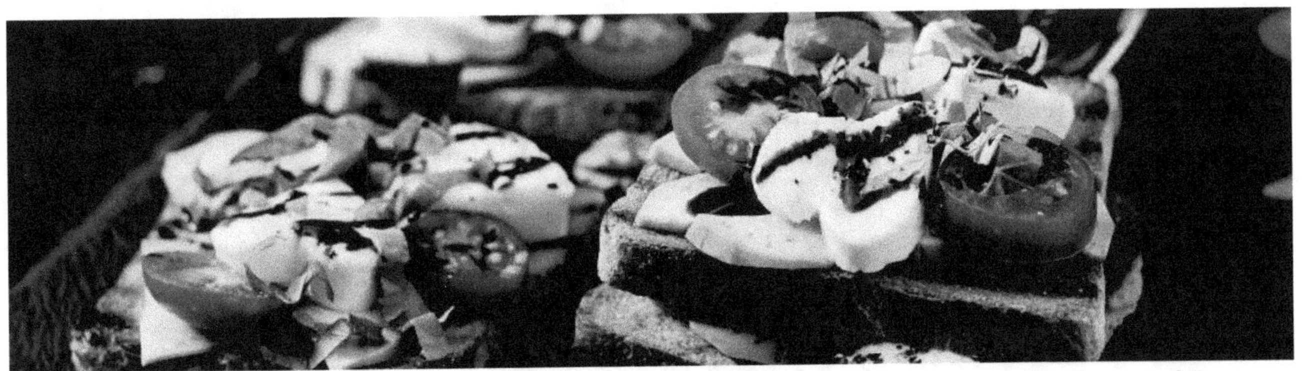

Avocado toast with tomato and basil

CALORIES: 228   **FAT: 17G**   **PROTEIN: 2.7G**   **CARB: 18G**

SERVINGS: 2   **PREP TIME: 5 MINS**   **TOTAL TIME: 5 MINS**

INGREDIENTS

2 pieces of french bread (or
bread of your choice).
1 large sliced hass avocado
1/2 cup chopped cherry tomatoes
3 cloves minced garlic
1 tablespoon olive oil, salt and
pepper to taste.
1 handful of fresh basil, rolled
and cut into strips.

DIRECTIONS

1. Place sliced avocado on toasted bread.
2. Toss the tomatoes with garlic, olive oil, salt, pepper, and basil.
3. Spoon on top of the avocado and dig in!

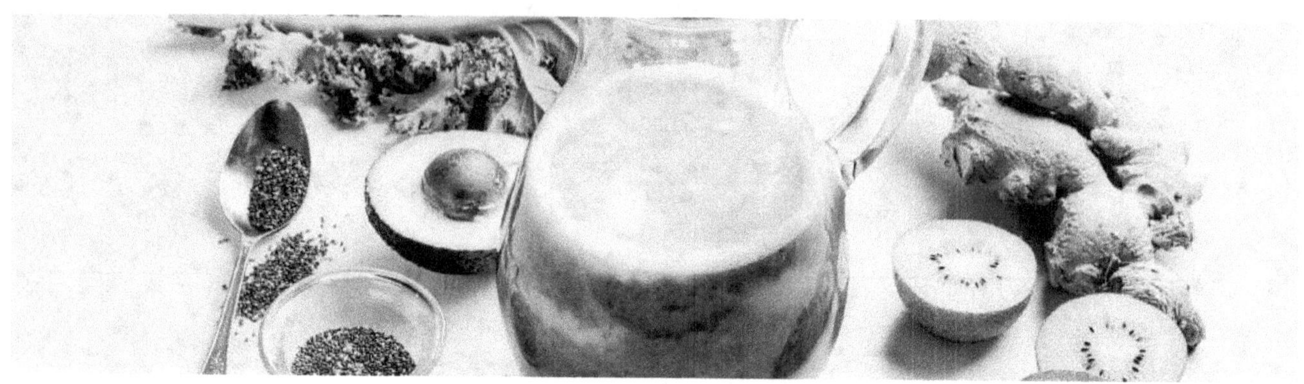

Green smoothie with kale, apple, and ginger

CALORIES: 347 **FAT: 5G** **PROTEIN: 32G** **CARB: 55G**

SERVINGS: 1 **PREP TIME: 5 MINS** **TOTAL TIME: 5 MINS**

INGREDIENTS

2 cups kale (loosely packed, stems removed).

1 medium apple (core removed, chopped into bits).

2 celery stalks (quartered)

½ large banana.

½ cup parsley

1 tablespoon of lemon juice.

1 inch of ginger root (quartered)

1 scoop of protein powder.

1 cup water.

Ice to taste.

DIRECTIONS

1. In a high-speed blender, combine all of the ingredients except the ice and purée until smooth. Add ice to taste, then pulse until creamy and smooth.

33

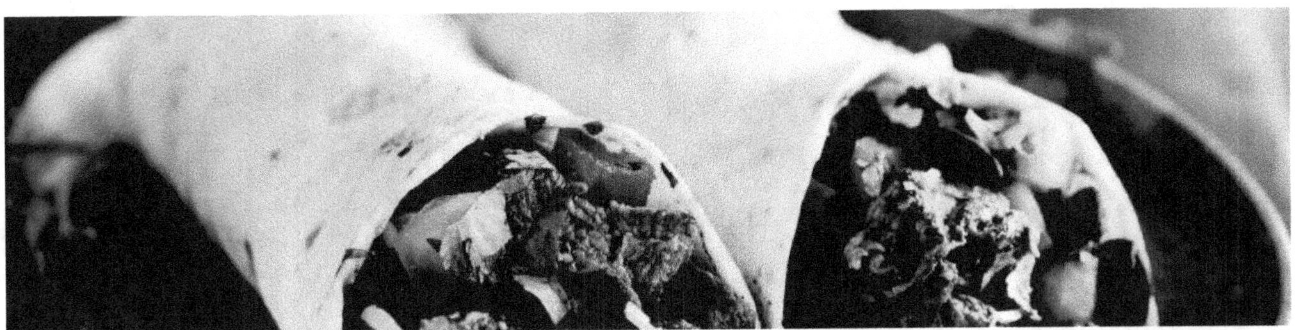

Breakfast burrito with black beans and salsa

CALORIES: 244   **FAT: 12G**   **PROTEIN: 17G**   **CARB: 18G**

SERVINGS: 1   **PREP TIME: 20 MINS**   **TOTAL TIME: 26 MINS**

INGREDIENTS

Ingredients: 2 tablespoons olive oil, 1 medium onion, 1 medium bell pepper, 15 ounces canned black beans (drained and rinsed), and 1/2 cup salsa.

½ teaspoon salt.

¼ teaspoon pepper.

¼ teaspoon cumin

¼ teaspoon paprika.

Six big eggs.

1/2 cup shredded Mexican cheese blend.

Six 8-inch tortillas.

DIRECTIONS

1. Add 1 tablespoon olive oil to a pan set over medium heat. Once heated, add the diced onion and bell pepper. Cook for 3-4 minutes, or until the onions start to turn translucent. Add the black beans, salsa, salt, pepper, cumin, and paprika, stirring to mix. Cook for another 2-3 minutes, then remove from the heat and put aside.

2. In a mixing dish, whisk together eggs. In a new nonstick skillet over medium-low heat, add 1 tablespoon olive oil. Pour in the eggs. As the eggs set on the bottom, use a spatula to pull them across the pan. This produces egg curds in the pan. Continue to pull and fold the eggs until no liquid remains. Remove from the heat and put aside. Allow the eggs to cool to room temperature to avoid adding too much moisture to the burritos.

3.......

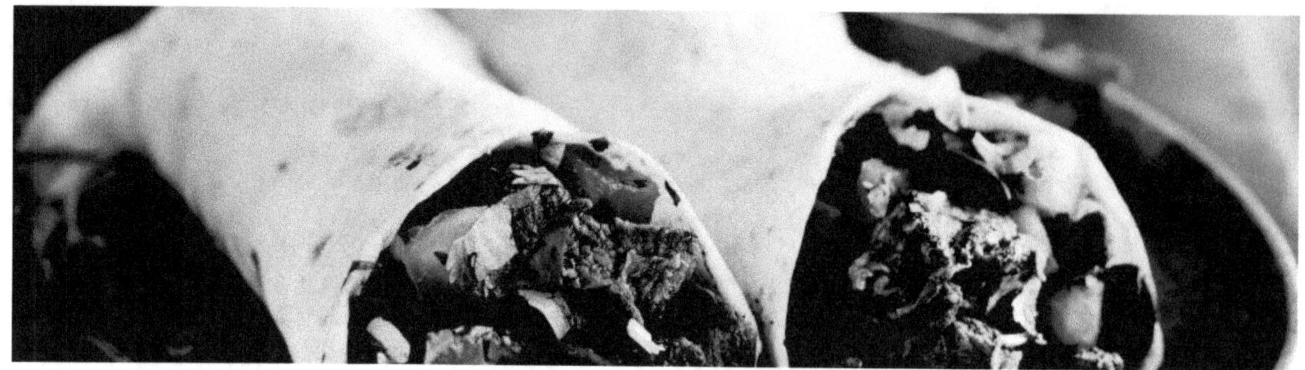

DIRECTIONS

3. Arrange 6 tortillas on top of 6 squares of foil. Place shredded cheese in the center of each tortilla. Then, divide the bean mixture evenly between the tortillas. Finally, divide your scrambled eggs amongst the tortillas. Wrap each tortilla tightly and then with foil.

4. Burritos should be stored in a gallon freezer bag or another freezer-safe container until they are ready to thaw and reheat.

Reheating Direction:

• Thaw the tortilla in the refrigerator overnight. In a nonstick pan over medium heat, cook the tortilla for 3-4 minutes on each side, or until it is browned and crispy. If the burrito is browning before the middle is warmed, reduce the heat slightly.

• Thawed or frozen, wrap the burrito in a moist paper towel and microwave for 1-2 minutes, or until heated thoroughly.

• Toaster oven/oven: Preheat to 350 degrees Fahrenheit and bake for 10 minutes for a thawed burrito or 15 minutes for a frozen burrito.

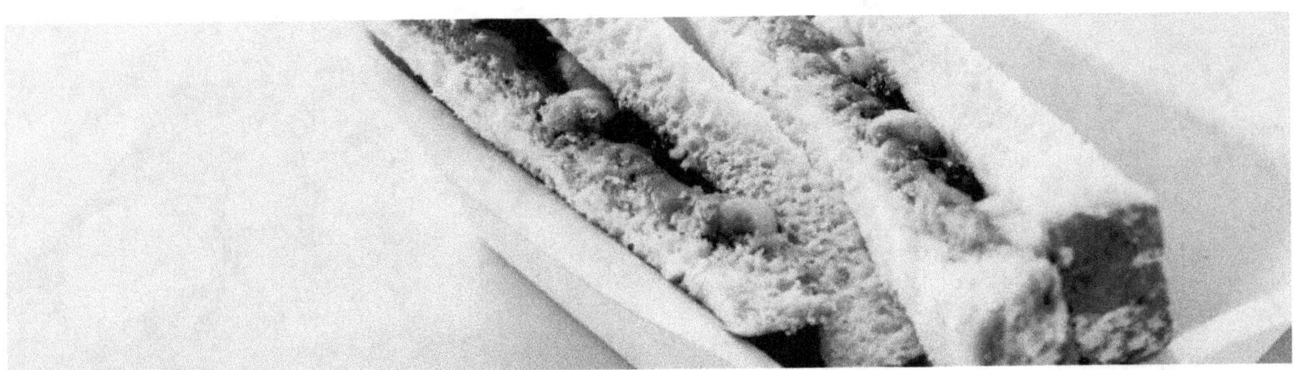

Peanut butter and banana sandwich

CALORIES: 299   **FAT: 9G**   **PROTEIN: 12G**   **CARB: 36G**

SERVINGS: 1   **PREP TIME: 2 MINS**   **TOTAL TIME: 10 MINS**

INGREDIENTS

2 pieces of 100% whole wheat bread with honey.
4 teaspoons of reduced-fat creamy peanut butter
One small banana or half of a medium banana, cut

DIRECTIONS

1. Toast the bread.
2. While the toast is still warm, put 2 teaspoons of peanut butter on each slice.
3. Place banana slices on one of the slices of peanut butter toast.
4. To make a sandwich, place the other piece on top, peanut butter side down.

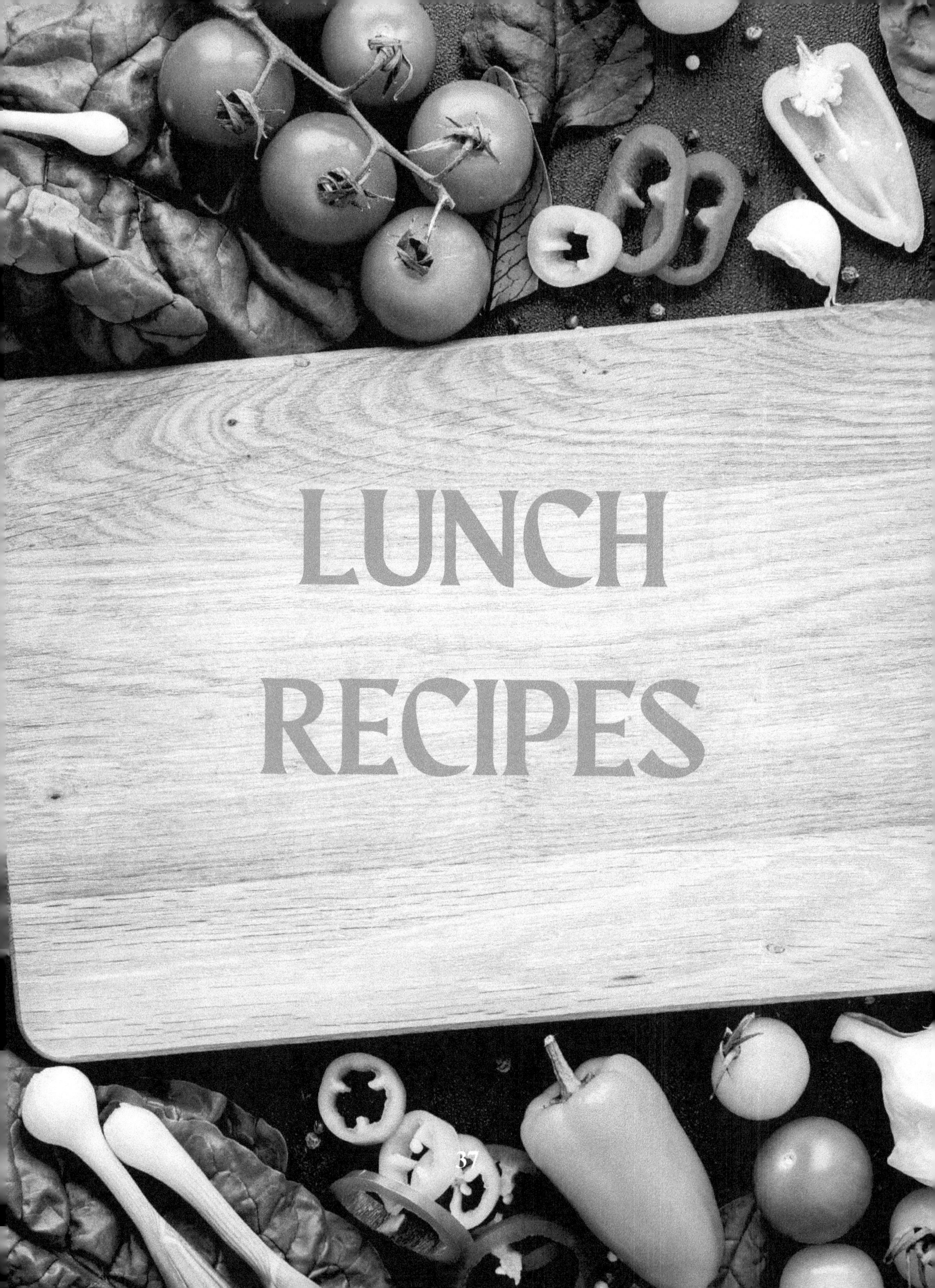

LUNCH
RECIPES
37

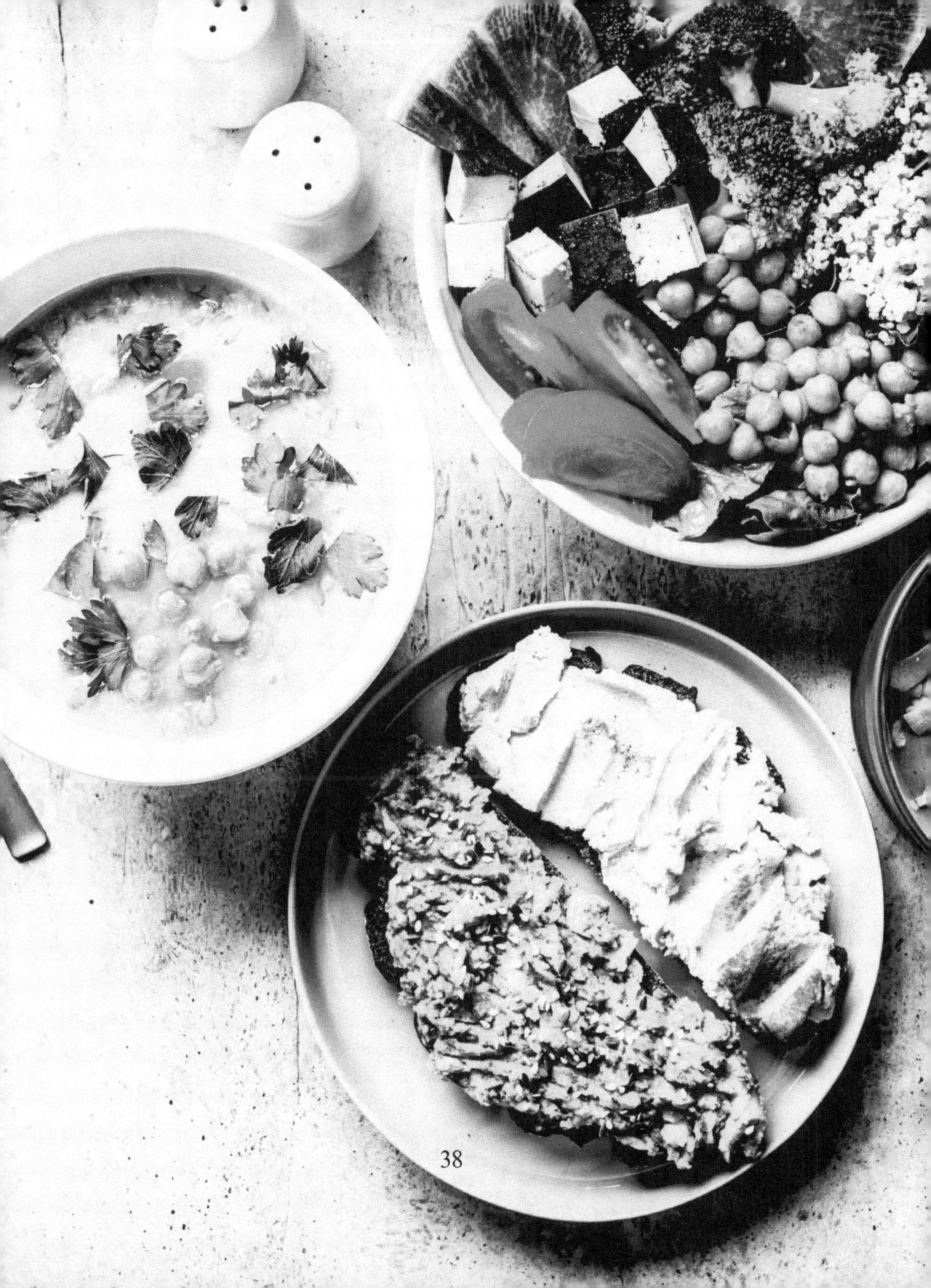

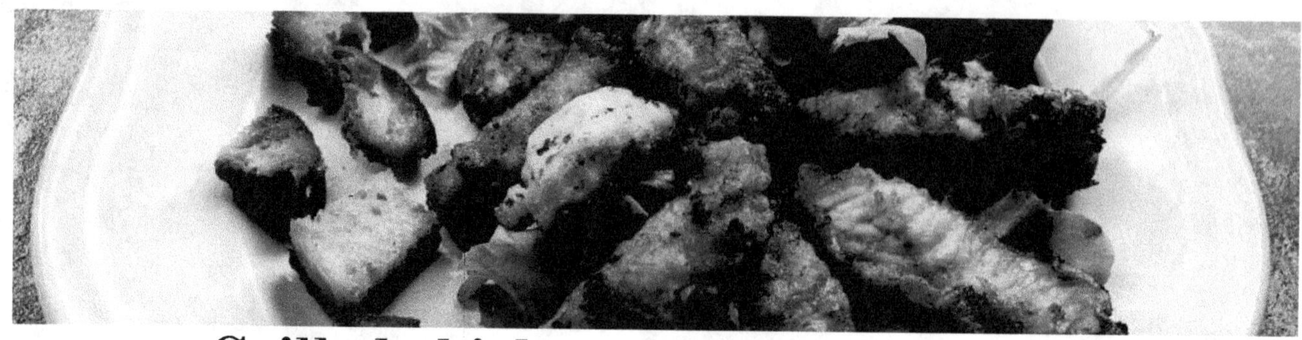

Grilled chicken salad with balsamic vinaigrette

CALORIES: 98 **FAT: 8G** **PROTEIN: 0.2G** **CARB: 7G**

SERVINGS: 1 **PREP TIME: 5 MINS** **COOK TIME: 20 MINS**

INGREDIENTS

Dress with 1/2 cup of
vintage balsamic vinegar.
1/2 cup apple cider vinegar.
Use 1/2 cup extra virgin
olive oil.
1/2 teaspoon garlic powder.
2 tablespoons of onion
powder.
1 teaspoon dry mustard.
1/2 teaspoon black pepper.
One teaspoon of salt.
4 Tbsp honey.

DIRECTIONS

1. Whisk thoroughly and chill in a pint jar.
Serve over salad with your desired
toppings.

> **Tips: Marinate one pound of chicken breast in two-thirds cup dressing overnight.**
> **Remove the chicken from the marinade and cook until 165 degrees Fahrenheit.**

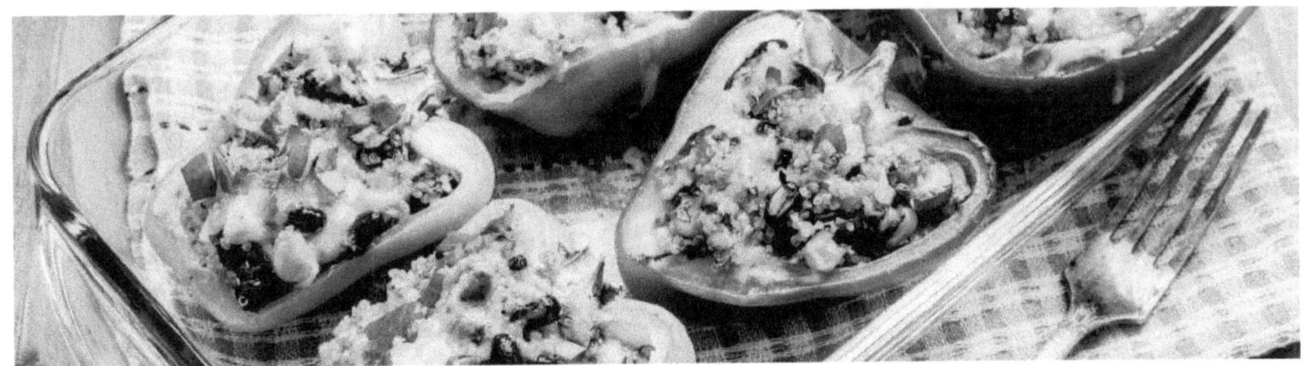

Quinoa-stuffed bell peppers

CALORIES: 286   **FAT: 5G**   **PROTEIN: 12G**   **CARB: 51G**

SERVINGS: 1   **PREP TIME: 10 MINS**   **COOK TIME: 40 MINS**

INGREDIENTS

6 medium bell peppers with tops cut off and cores removed.
1 cup uncooked quinoa, rinsed and drained
Combine 2 cups vegetable broth with 1 tablespoon olive oil.
Chop one small onion and mince two garlic cloves.
1 15-ounce can of chopped tomatoes
1 15-ounce can of black beans.
1 cup frozen corn (thawed)
One teaspoon cumin.
One teaspoon of paprika.
Combine ½ teaspoon salt and ¼ teaspoon black pepper.
1 cup freshly grated Monterey Jack cheese.
Optional toppings include chopped fresh cilantro, cubed avocado, and sour cream.

DIRECTIONS

1. Place the quinoa and vegetable broth in a medium saucepan. Bring the mixture to a boil over medium-high heat. Reduce the heat to a simmer, cover, and cook for 15 minutes, or until the liquid is fully absorbed. Allow the quinoa to sit for 5 minutes without opening the cover before fluffing with a fork.

2. Preheat the oven to 375° Fahrenheit. Cut the peppers in half lengthwise, then take off the seeds and membrane. Place the peppers cut side up in a baking dish, then add enough water to cover the bottom.

3. .....

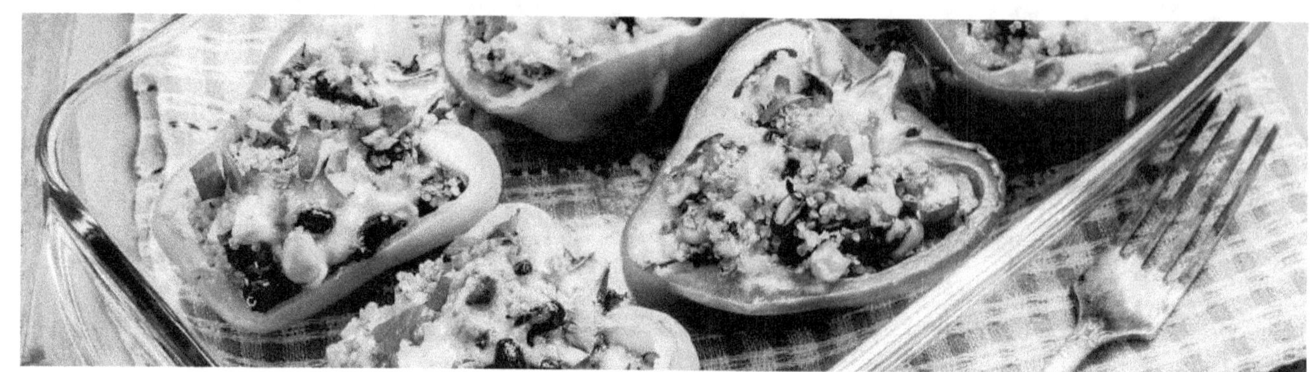

DIRECTIONS

3. In a large nonstick skillet, heat the olive oil over medium heat. Sauté the onions for 2-3 minutes, or until they soften slightly. Add the garlic and cook for another minute, or until fragrant. Combine the cooked quinoa, diced tomatoes, black beans, and corn. Season with cumin, paprika, salt, and pepper. Reduce the heat to low and simmer for an additional 5 minutes, stirring frequently.

4. Carefully spoon the mixture into the sliced peppers, then sprinkle with cheese.

5. Bake uncovered for 30-35 minutes, or until the peppers are tender and the cheese has melted. Add optional toppings and serve hot.

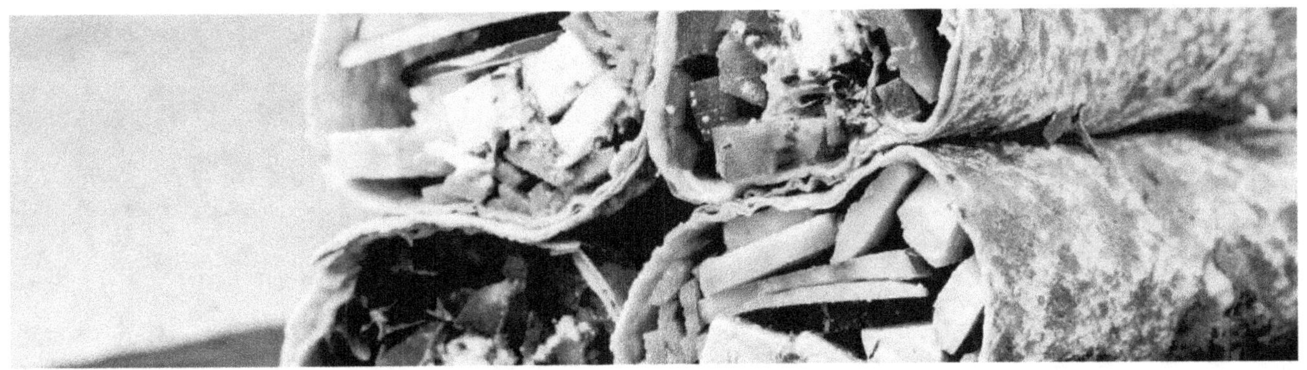

Whole Wheat Vegetable Wrap with Hummus

CALORIES: 345   **FAT: 17G**   **PROTEIN: 11G**   **CARB: 38G**

SERVINGS: 1   **PREP TIME: 10 MINS**   **TOTAL TIME: 10 MINS**

INGREDIENTS

One 8-inch whole wheat
tortilla.
2 tablespoons hummus.
¼ avocado mashed
1 cup sliced, fresh
vegetables of your choice.
2 tablespoons shredded
strong cheddar cheese.

DIRECTIONS

1. Lay the tortilla on the work surface. Spread hummus and avocado onto a tortilla. Roll up the veggies and cheddar cheese. Divide in half before serving.

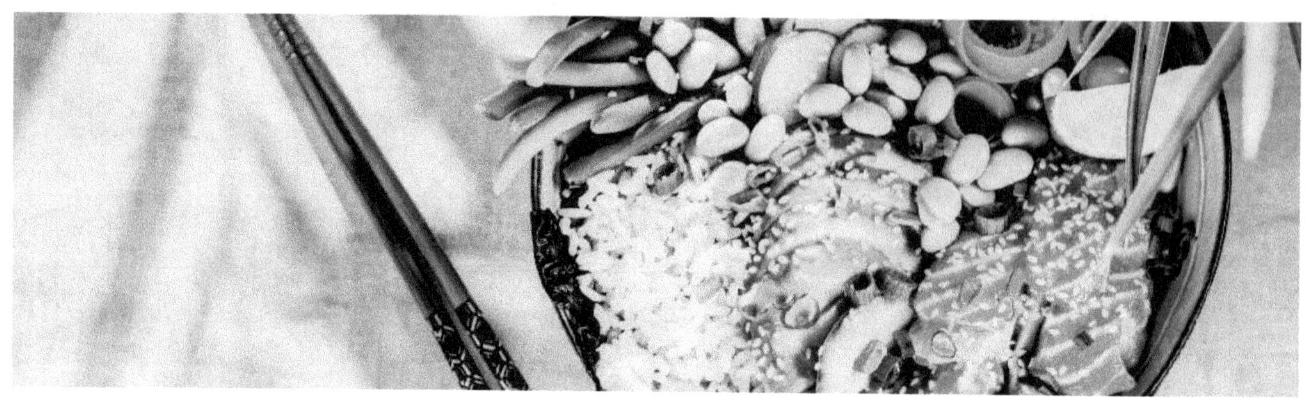

Salmon and Avocado Sushi Bowl

CALORIES: 439 **FAT: 1.3G** **PROTEIN: 21G** **CARB: 67G**

SERVINGS: 4 **PREP TIME: 20 MINS** **COOK TIME: 15 MINS**

INGREDIENTS

215g (1 cup) sushi rice and 60mL (1/4 cup) sushi seasoning
200 g frozen edamame.
200g snow peas, trimmed
Ingredients: 1 large avocado, quartered 185g hot-smoked salmon (skin removed and flaked).
Two carrots were peeled and sliced into ribbons.
Strip two Lebanese cucumbers into ribbons.
1/4 nori sheet, finely shredded
Two teaspoons of wasabi peas.
To serve, use Kewpie mayonnaise.
To serve, add soy sauce.

DIRECTIONS

1. Place the rice and 375ml (1 1/2 cups) water in a saucepan over medium heat. Bring to a boil, stirring occasionally. Reduce the heat to low. Cover and cook for 10-15 minutes, until the water is absorbed. Set aside, covered, for 5 minutes. Transfer the rice to a large bowl. Drizzle the sushi seasoning over the rice, then fold with a large spoon until well combined. Set aside to cool.

2.........

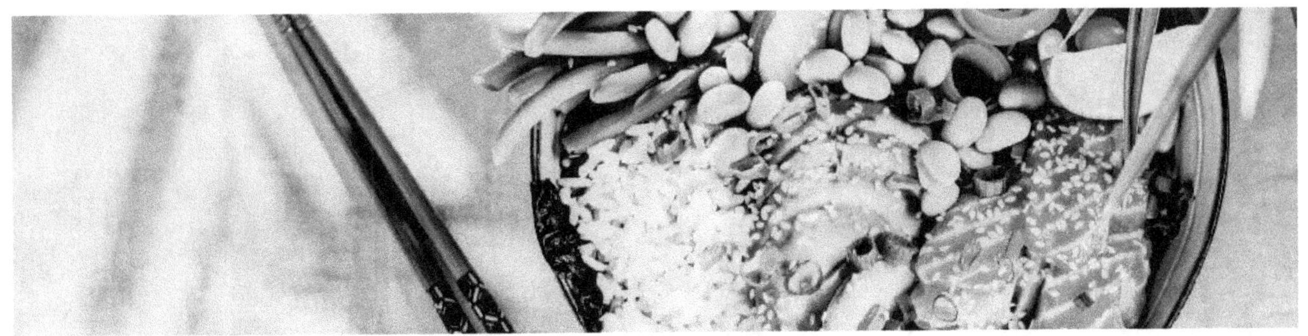

DIRECTIONS

2. Meanwhile, in a small saucepan of boiling water, cook the edamame for 3 minutes until mushy. Refresh with cool running water. Drain. Remove the edamame pods and place them in a basin. Discard the pods. Place the snow peas in a heat-resistant container and cover with boiling water. Set aside for 1 minute. Drain and chill in a basin of ice water. Drain. Pat the snow peas dry before cutting them into long, thin strips

3. Divide the rice among the serving bowls. Top with avocado, salmon, carrots, cucumbers, snow peas, and edamame. Sprinkle with shredded nori and wasabi peas. Squeeze some mayonnaise over the rice. Pour soy sauce over the avocado.

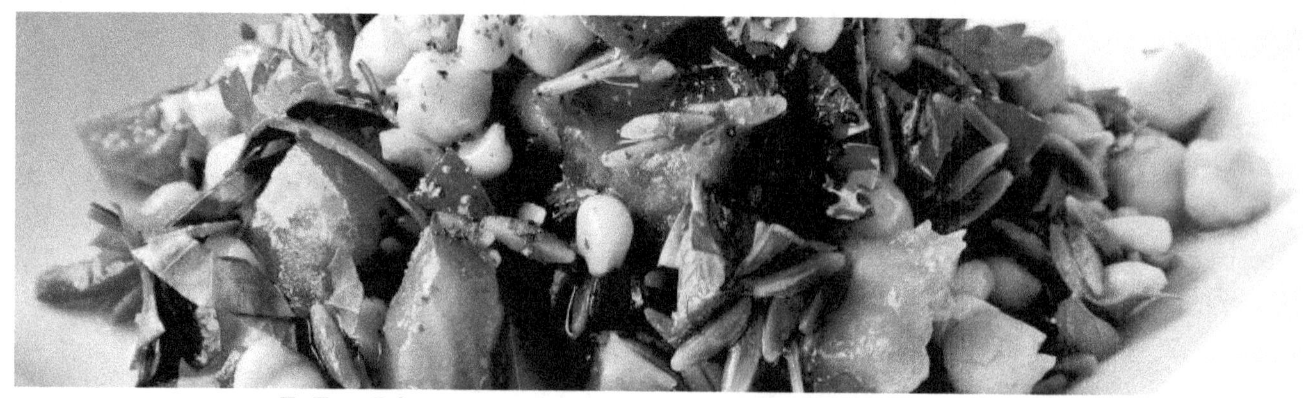

Mediterranean chickpea salad

CALORIES: 174   **FAT: 14.4G**   **PROTEIN: 2.5G**   **CARB: 12.1G**

SERVINGS: 6   **PREP TIME: 10 MINS**   **TOTAL TIME: 10 MINS**

INGREDIENTS

FOR THE DIJON DRESSING.
One teaspoon Dijon mustard.
One lemon juice.
One garlic clove, minced
One teaspoon of Aleppo pepper.
One teaspoon of sumac.
Kosher salt.
Combine black pepper
and ¼ cup extra virgin olive oil.
FOR THE SALAD:
Two (15-ounce) cans of chickpeas, drained and rinsed
Chop one large English cucumber and halve two cups of grape tomatoes.
2 roasted red peppers, seeded and diced (or a 16-ounce container of oil-roasted peppers).
One small red onion or two shallots, coarsely chopped
1 cup chopped parsley leaves.
1/2 cup chopped mint leaves.
An avocado, pitted and roughly cut

DIRECTIONS

1. Make some dressing. In a large bowl, combine Dijon, lemon juice, garlic, Aleppo pepper, sumac, salt, and pepper (approximately ½ teaspoon each). Whisk, then sprinkle with enough olive oil to make it glossy and well-balanced. Continue to whisk until emulsified.
2. Mix. In a bowl, mix the chickpeas, cucumbers, tomatoes, roasted bell peppers, onion, parsley, and mint with the vinaigrette. Toss softly.
3. Add the avocado and toss gently once more.
4. Enjoy! Taste, adjust the seasoning, and serve immediately.

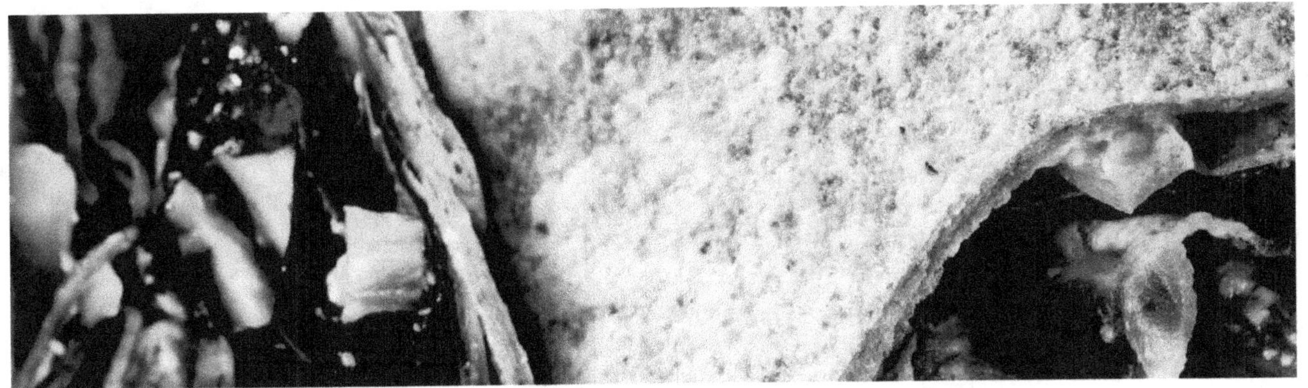

Pesto Roasted Vegetable Wrap

CALORIES: 592.53   **FAT: 47G**   **PROTEIN: 14G**   **CARB: 31G**

SERVINGS: 3   **PREP TIME: 20 MINS**   **TOTAL TIME: 50 MINS**

INGREDIENTS

6 cups of mixed vegetables.
Ingredients: ¼ cup balsamic
vinegar and ¼ cup olive oil
1 teaspoon Italian herbs, or
mix together rosemary,
thyme, oregano, and/or
marjoram.
Three flour tortillas.
3 oz goat cheese.
For Pesto:
1 cup of fresh basil leaves
(around 4 ounces)
1/2 cup pine nuts.
2 tablespoons olive oil
1 tablespoon parmesan
cheese, shredded
One garlic clove.

DIRECTIONS

PESTO:

1. Put everything in a food processor and pulse for approximately a minute, until a vibrant green paste forms.

ROAST THE VEGETABLES:

2. Preheat the oven to 450 °F.

3. Place the vegetables, vinegar, olive oil, and herbs in the storage container. Snap the top and shake to coat the vegetables.

4. Allow to marinate for 5–10 minutes.

5. Pour the vegetables and marinade onto a baking sheet and spread them out in one layer.

6. Roast for 10 minutes. Toss the vegetables around with tongs, then roast for a further 10 minutes.

7. The edges should be black. Turn off the oven and use the oven mitts to remove the baking sheet.

8. ....

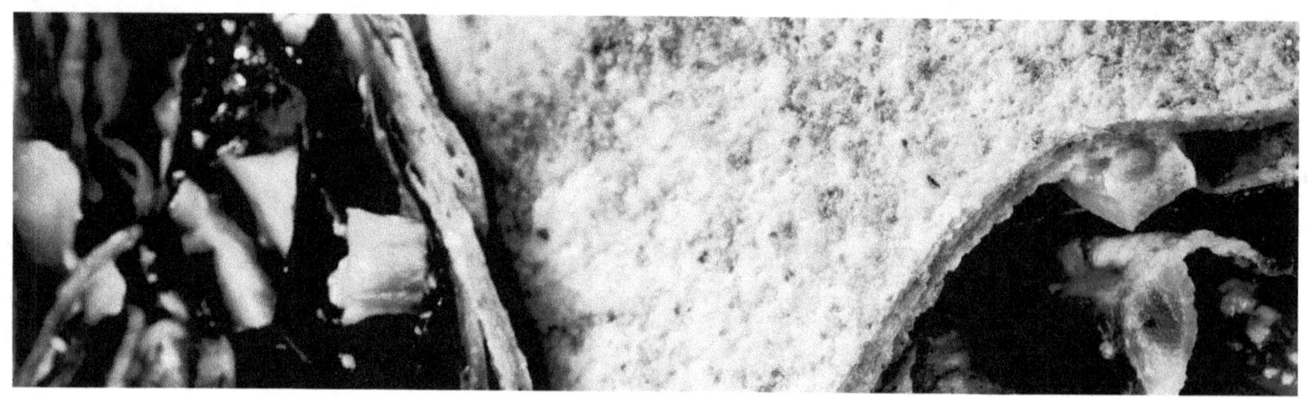

DIRECTIONS

TO ASSEMBLE:

9. Spread 1 tablespoon pesto on each tortilla, then divide the vegetables between them. Top with dollops of goat cheese and roll up.

10. Serve and enjoy!

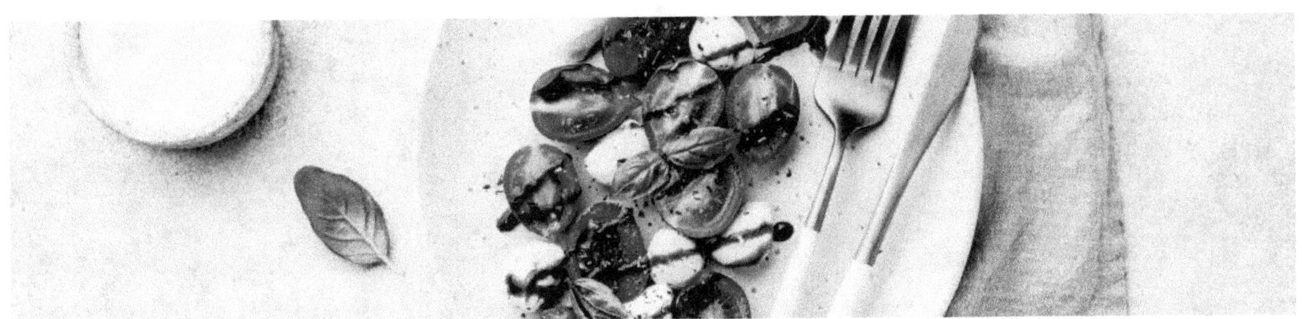

Caprese salad features mozzarella, tomatoes, and basil

CALORIES: 245　　**FAT: 17G**　　**PROTEIN: 15G**　　**CARB: 11G**

SERVINGS: 4　　**PREP TIME: 10 MINS**　　**TOTAL TIME: 10 MINS**

INGREDIENTS

1 1/2 to 2 pounds of heirloom tomatoes, cored and sliced 1/4 to 1/3 inch thick (a serrated knife is best for this).
Kosher or sea salt?
1 bunch of fresh basil, with the leaves properly chopped or torn to avoid bruises.
8 ounces of fresh mozzarella cheese, sliced
One tablespoon of extra virgin olive oil.
A dash of balsamic vinegar is optional.
Fresh ground black pepper.

DIRECTIONS

1. Sprinkle salt lightly over the tomato slices.
2. To create the salad, alternate pieces of tomato, basil leaves, and mozzarella.
3. Drizzle the salad with extra virgin olive oil. If using, mix in a little bit of balsamic vinegar. Season lightly with pepper.

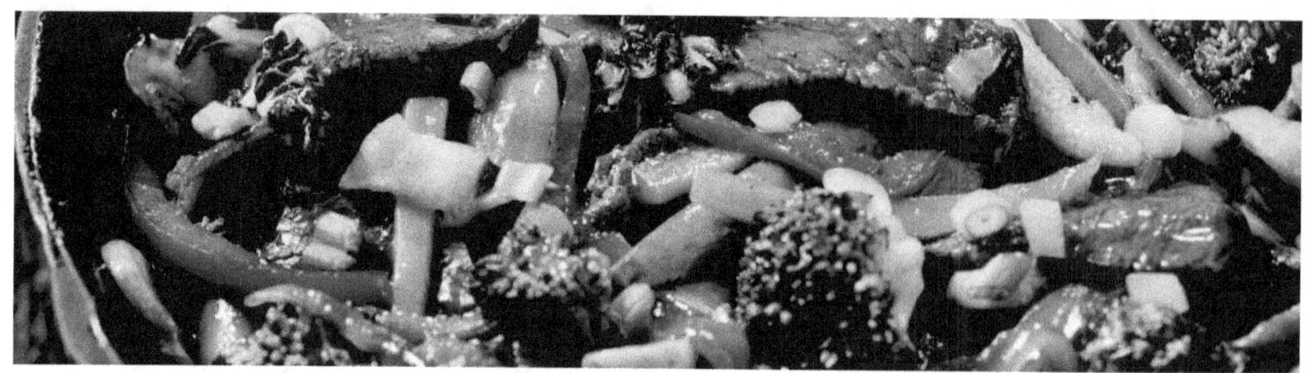

Vegetable Stir-Fry with Tofu

CALORIES: 334   **FAT: 21G**   **PROTEIN: 12G**   **CARB: 25G**

SERVINGS: 1   **PREP TIME: 25 MINS**   **COOL TIME: 15 MINS**

INGREDIENTS

3-4 tablespoons of neutral-flavored high-heat oil (e.g., avocado oil)

Tofu:

Use 1 (14-ounce/400g) block of extra-firm tofu, preferably frozen and defrosted
½ teaspoon kosher salt
½ teaspoon white pepper
½ teaspoon garlic powder, and 1/4 teaspoon Chinese five spice powder (optional but wonderful!).
Combine 3 tablespoons cornstarch or arrowroot powder.
To prepare stir fry sauce, mix 1 ½ teaspoons soy sauce (tamari for gluten-free)
1 ½ tablespoons rice vinegar
2 tablespoons of hoisin sauce, and 2 tablespoons of Shaoxing wine (Chinese cooking wine) (see Note 3 for substitutes).
1 tablespoon organic brown sugar
Add 1-2 teaspoons of chili-garlic sauce (or sambal oelek) (2 for spicy!)
Add 3 tbsp veggie broth/water

Continuation ■

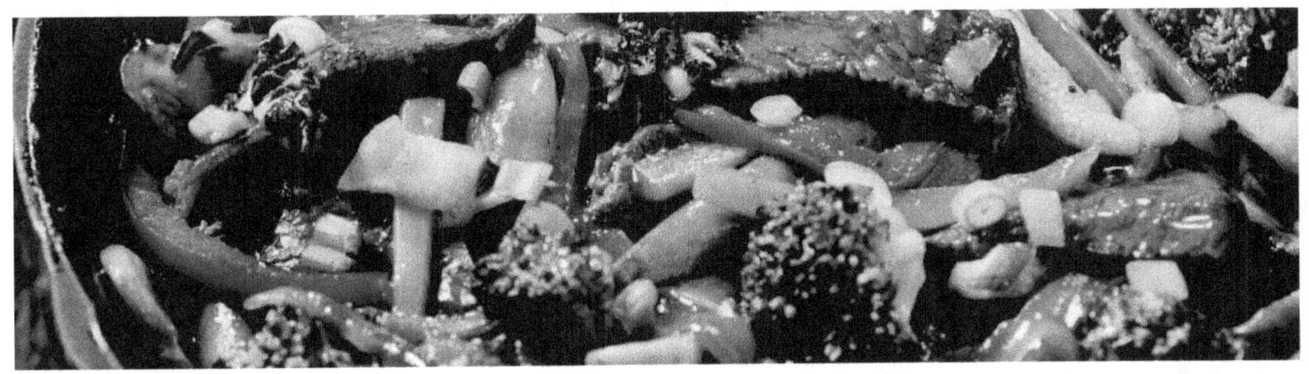

INGREDIENTS

Aromatic and Vegetables

2 inches finely chopped ginger (not grated or minced)
4 cloves of chopped garlic (not minced)
14-16 oz vegetables of your choosing.
To finish, combine 1 teaspoon cornstarch (or arrowroot powder) and 1 tablespoon cold water.
To prepare, combine 2 teaspoons black or toasted white sesame seeds
2 teaspoons toasted sesame oil
¾ cup (12g) finely cut cilantro leaves and delicate stems
3 to 4 cups of cooked white or brown rice for serving.

DIRECTIONS

1. Drain the tofu and wrap in a thin dish towel. Weight down with a heavy cookbook or skillet. Press for 10-15 minutes, changing the towel midway. Meanwhile, mix the Sauce ingredients in a bowl or measuring cup while preparing the veggies and aromatics.
2. Cut the tofu. Cut the tofu in four equal squares. After flipping each square on its side, cut into ⅓" (~1 cm) squares and place in a large basin or shallow baking pan.
3. Coat the tofu. In a small bowl, combine the salt, white pepper, garlic powder, five spice powder (if using), and cornstarch. Sprinkle half of the mixture over the tofu, flip it over, and then sprinkle with the remaining ingredients, gently tossing to coat.
4. ....

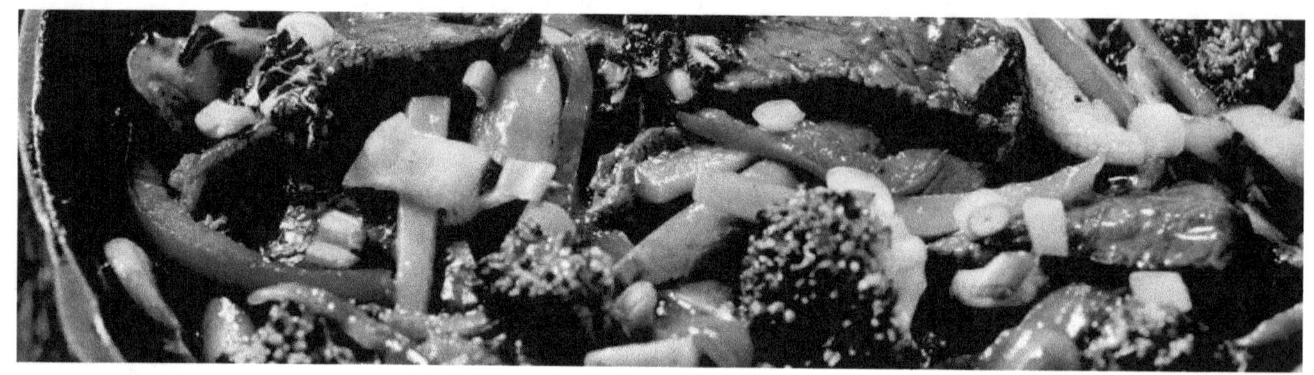

DIRECTIONS

4. To fry the tofu, line a chopping board or large dish with paper towels, and open the windows if you're cooking in a wok, as it will smoke.

5. Heat a flat-bottomed wok over medium-high heat until you see small wisps of smoke, then add 3 tablespoons of oil (to prevent sticking), swirling the pan to spread the oil up the sides.

6. Cook the tofu for 3 to 5 minutes, shaking the pan every minute to ensure even cooking, until golden brown on the bottom. Flip and stir the tofu, then cook for 2 to 4 minutes, until golden brown but not burned on the bottom. Transfer the tofu to a paper towel-lined surface to absorb any excess oil, and wipe the pan.

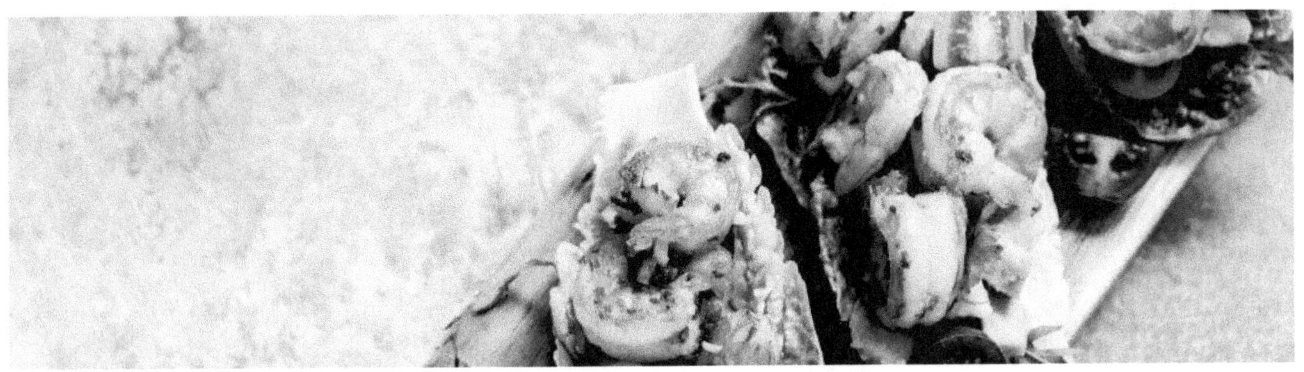

Shrimp tacos with cilantro-lime slaw

CALORIES: 2151   **FAT: 136G**   **PROTEIN: 93G**   **CARB: 164G**

SERVINGS: 8   **PREP TIME: 15 MINS**   **TOTAL TIME: 8 MINS**

INGREDIENTS

Regarding the shrimp tacos:

1 1/2 pounds jumbo shrimp, cooked, peeled, and deveined.

2 teaspoons chili powder.

2 tablespoons ground cumin

1/2 teaspoon onion powder.

1/2 teaspoon of garlic powder.

1/4 teaspoon of cayenne pepper.

1/2 teaspoon of salt.

Juice from 1/2 lime

One teaspoon of oil.

8 corn tortillas.

DIRECTIONS

1. Dry the shrimp with paper towels, then toss them in a medium bowl with the spice mixture and half a lime juice until thoroughly incorporated.

2. Heat the oil in a large skillet over medium-high heat, then add the shrimp and cook for 5-8 minutes, flipping frequently, until fully cooked.

3. ......

Continuation ■

52

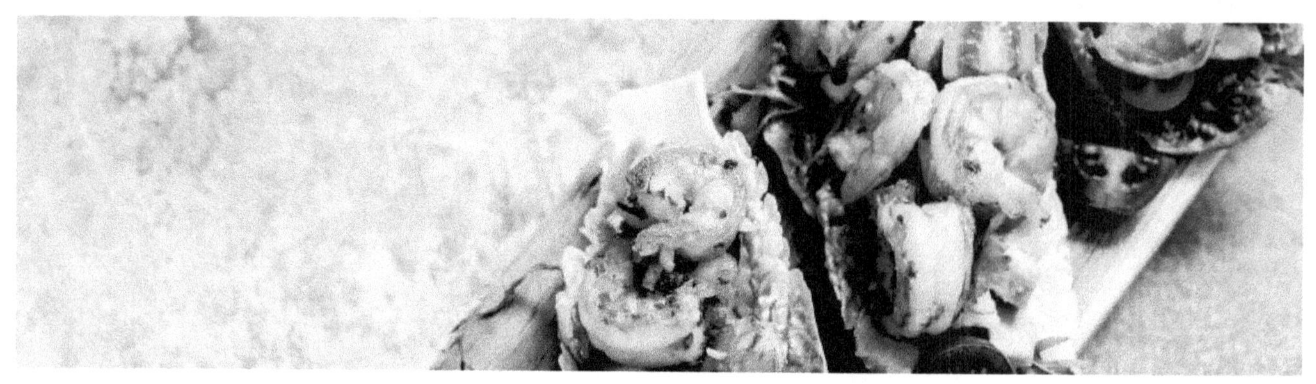

INGREDIENTS

For coleslaw:

2 cups shredded green cabbage.
2 cups shredded purple cabbage.
1 cup shredded carrots.
1/4 cup chopped fresh cilantro.
Add 2 tablespoons of lime juice
(about 1-2 tablespoons).
Ingredients include 1 tablespoon,
1/4 teaspoon salt, and freshly
ground pepper.

Optional toppings:

Avocado, cotija cheese, more
cilantro, and lime juice

DIRECTIONS

3. In a large mixing bowl, combine all
of the slaw ingredients.

4. Layer mashed avocado, shrimp, and
slaw on warm corn tortillas, then top
with cheese, fresh cilantro, and lime
juice if desired

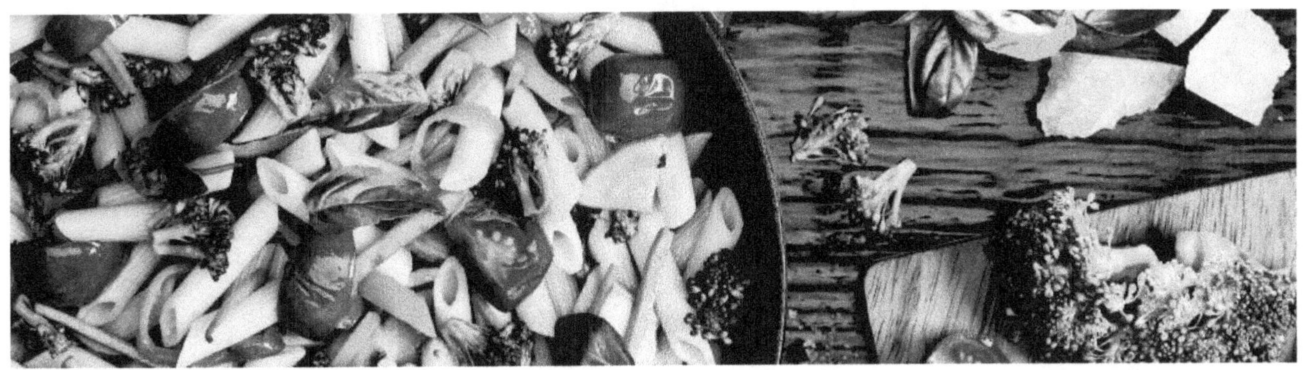

Pasta primavera using whole wheat pasta

CALORIES: 229 **FAT: 9G** **PROTEIN: 9G** **CARB: 33G**

SERVINGS: 6 **PREP TIME: 20 MINS** **TOTAL TIME: 40 MINS**

INGREDIENTS

3 carrots, peeled and sliced
2 yellow squash, sliced
1 onion, thinly sliced
1 yellow bell pepper, cut into strips.
One red bell pepper, cut into strips.
1 head broccoli, cut into florets,
with stems chopped.
Combine 1/4 cup olive oil, salt, and
freshly ground black pepper.
1 tablespoon dried Italian
seasoning.
1 tablespoon of garlic powder (to
taste)
Crushed red pepper flakes are
optional.
One pound whole wheat pasta.
15 cherry tomatoes, half.
Ingredients: 1/2 cup grated
Parmesan or Romano cheese, more
cheese for serving, and optional
shredded fresh basil.

DIRECTIONS

1. Preheat your oven to 450 degrees.
2. Toss the veggies (excluding the cherry tomatoes) in a large bowl with the olive oil, salt, pepper, Italian spices, garlic powder, and crushed red pepper, if desired.
3. Place the vegetables on two large baking sheets, ensuring a homogeneous layer.
4. Bake until the carrots are tender and the other vegetables start to brown and caramelize.
5. After around 10 minutes of cooking, quickly mix the vegetables.
6. Boil salted water and cook the pasta
7. .....

54

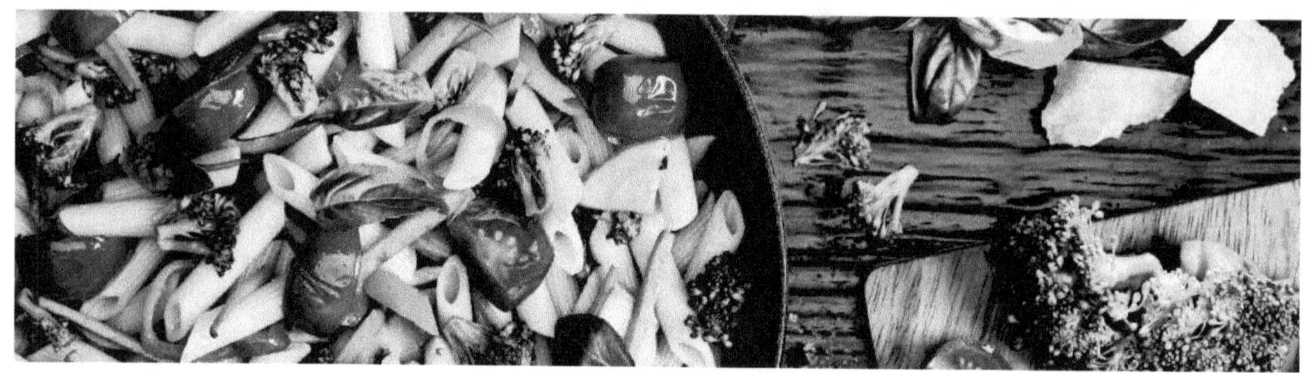

DIRECTIONS

8. Drain the pasta and reserve about a cup of the cooking liquid

9. Combine the pasta and vegetables in a large bowl.

10. If the pasta appears too dry, add the cherry tomatoes and any remaining cooking liquid.

11. Season with salt and pepper to taste.

12. Sprinkle with your preferred shredded cheese and fresh basil leaves.

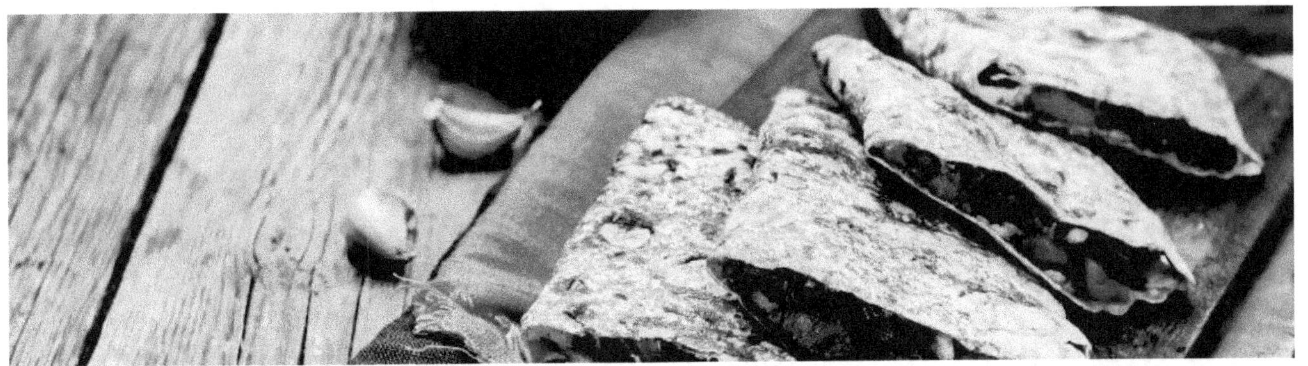

Black bean and sweet potato quesadillas

CALORIES: 663   **FAT: 17G**   **PROTEIN: 26G**   **CARB: 103G**

SERVINGS: 4   **PREP TIME: 15 MINS**   **COOK TIME: 35 MINS**

INGREDIENTS

One large sweet potato, peeled
and chopped
1 tablespoon chopped fresh
cilantro
¼ teaspoon chili powder.
½ teaspoon salt
¼ cup frozen corn.
1 (19-ounce) can of black beans,
drained and rinsed
Eight (8 inch) flour tortillas.
1 cup shredded cheddar cheese.
Cooking Spray

DIRECTIONS

1. Place the sweet potatoes in a big pot and fill with salted water. Bring to the boil. Reduce heat to medium-low and simmer for 15 minutes, or until very tender. Drain and transfer to a bowl. Mash sweet potatoes and add cilantro, chili powder, and salt.

2. Place corn in a microwave-safe bowl and heat on high for 1 to 2 minutes.

3. Spread 1/4 cup sweet potato mixture on one tortilla; top with 1/4 cup black beans and 1 tablespoon corn. Sprinkle 1/4 cup Cheddar cheese over the corn and wrap with a tortilla. Repeat with the remaining tortillas and contents.

4. Spray a frying pan with cooking spray and place it over medium heat; cook 1 quesadilla until the cheese melts and the beans are heated through, about 3 to 4 minutes per side. Repeat with the remaining quesadillas; cut into quarters.

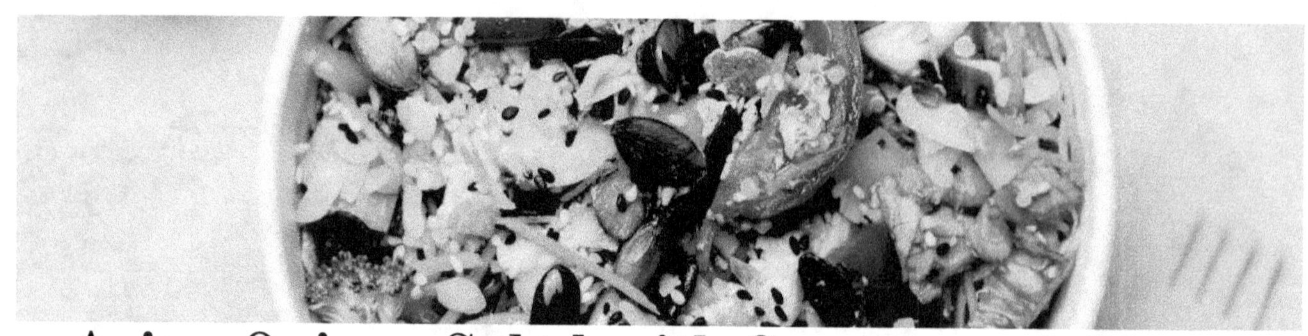

Asian Quinoa Salad with Sesame and Ginger Dressing

CALORIES: 224   **FAT: 5G**   **PROTEIN: 10G**   **CARB: 37G**

SERVINGS: 6   **PREP TIME: 15 MINS**   **TOTAL TIME: 15 MINS**

INGREDIENTS

Quinoa Salad.

1 cup shelled and boiled edamame
(124g)
1 cup diced cucumber,
approximately 128g.
1 cup sliced bell peppers (100g)
4 cups of Bob's Red Mill Organic
Tri-Color Quinoa, cooked
1 big shredded carrot or around 1
cup (67g/cup)
1 ½ cups chopped cabbage (100g)

Sesame Ginger Dressing

½ teaspoon ground ginger.
1 ½ tbsp. maple syrup.
2 ½ tablespoons liquid amino or
low-sodium soy sauce
2 teaspoons of distilled white
vinegar.
1 teaspoon of sesame oil.
1/2 teaspoon sesame seeds.
¼ teaspoon red pepper flakes
(optional)
Juice from two limes

DIRECTIONS

Sesame Ginger Dressing

1. Whisk all of the ingredients
together in a large mixing bowl until
well incorporated, or shake in a jar.
Set away until ready for use.

Asian Quinoa Salad

2. Mix all of the ingredients together
in a bowl.

3. Drizzle the sauce over the salad
and toss to incorporate.

4. Serve, and enjoy!

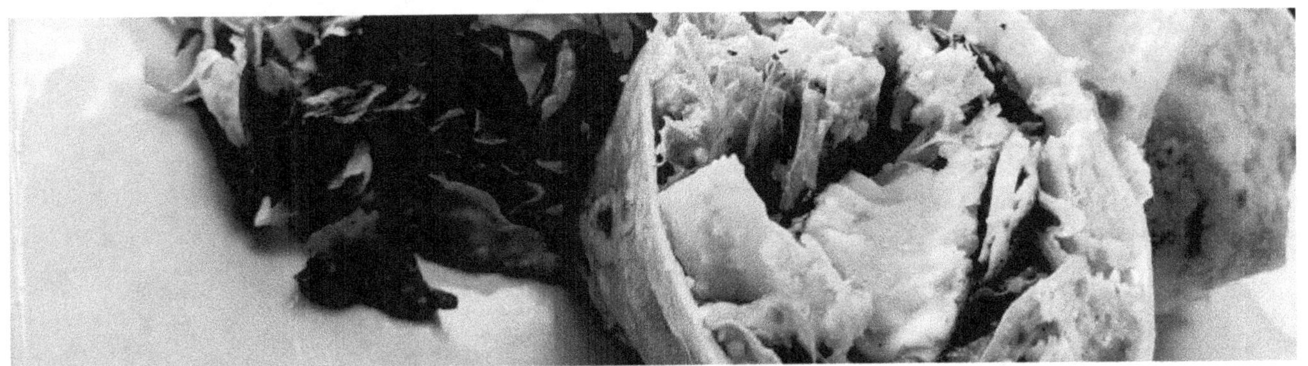

Chicken Caesar wraps with Romaine lettuce

CALORIES: 249　　　**FAT: 29G**　　　**PROTEIN: 35G**　　　**CARB: 50G**

SERVINGS: 5　　　**PREP TIME: 10 MINS**　　　**TOTAL TIME: 10 MINS**

INGREDIENTS

3 and 1/2 cups cooked chicken (I used rotisserie chicken to save time)

1/2 - 3/4 cup Caesar salad dressing (I prefer this one or my Greek yogurt one)

1/4 cup grated Parmesan cheese.

1/4 cup shredded radicchio.

Fresh lemon juice, squeezed

1/4 cup of smashed gluten-free croutons, crackers, or cheese crisps

Serve in romaine lettuce cups.

DIRECTIONS

1. In a large mixing bowl, combine the ingredients. I like to use less dressing to start since you can add as much as you like.
2. Layer two leaves on top of each other to form each wrap.
3. Add scoops of chicken salad on lettuce and serve.

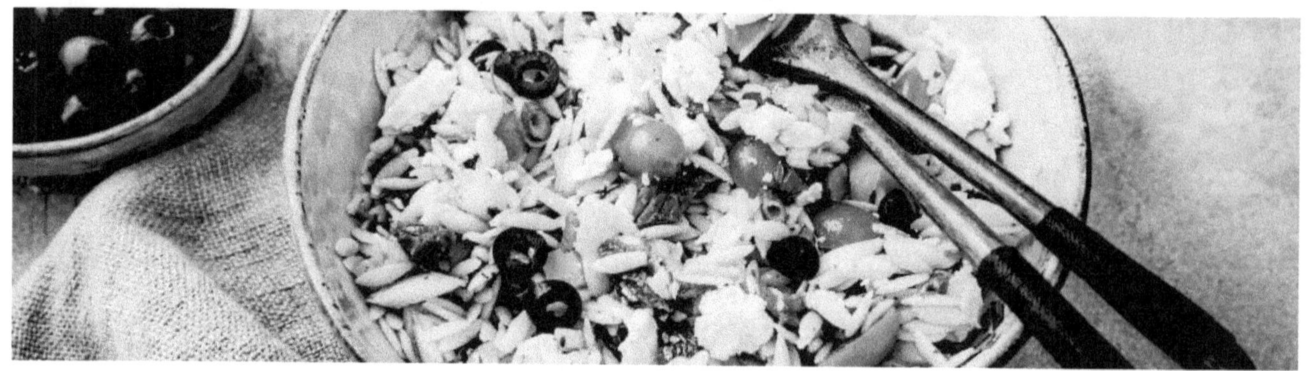

Greek orzo salad with feta and olives

CALORIES: 320   **FAT: 19G**   **PROTEIN: 8G**   **CARB: 28G**

SERVINGS: 6   **PREP TIME: 20 MINS**   **TOTAL TIME: 10 MINS**

INGREDIENTS

Dressing

1/3 cup olive oil.
3 tablespoons fresh lemon juice
1 clove garlic, minced
salt and freshly ground black pepper.

Salad

1 1/4 cups (8 oz) dried orzo
One cup (5 ounces) crumbled feta
One medium English cucumber, diced
1 (10.5 ounce) package. Grape
tomatoes halved
1/2 cup sliced Kalamata olives (or 3/4
cup sliced Black olives)
1/2 cup chopped red onion.
3 tablespoons chopped fresh basil
3 tablespoons chopped fresh parsley.

DIRECTIONS

1. In a medium mixing bowl, combine olive oil, lemon juice, and garlic; season with salt and pepper to taste. Set aside.

2. Cook the orzo according to the package directions until al dente, or just 1 minute shy. Drain and rinse with cold water for approximately 10 seconds. Drain well.

3. Toss all of the salad ingredients together in a big basin, including the cooked orzo. Toss the salad with the dressing to coat evenly.

4. Store in the refrigerator for up to two days.

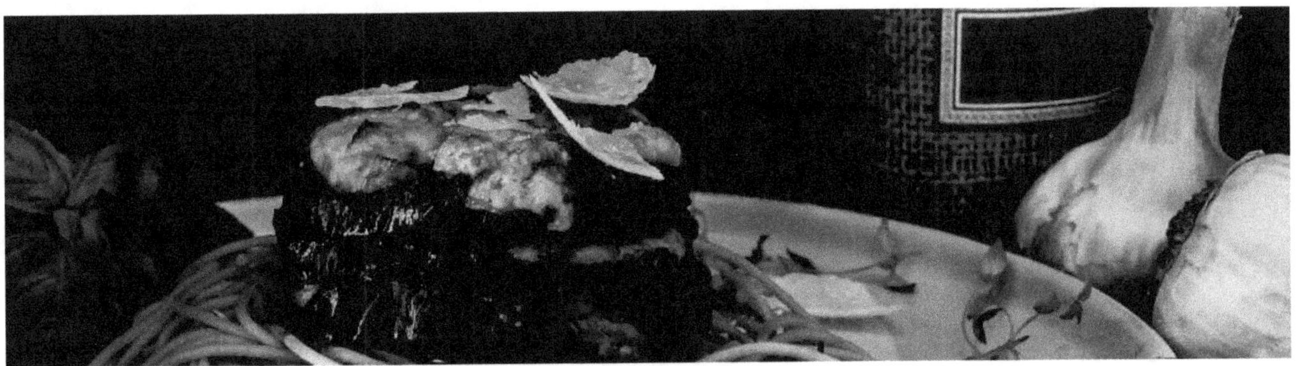

Eggplant Parmesan with Whole Grain Pasta

CALORIES: 370   **FAT: 10G**   **PROTEIN: 22G**   **CARB: 56G**

SERVINGS: 6   **PREP TIME: 15 MINS**   **COOK TIME: 15 MINS**

INGREDIENTS

12 ounces whole grain spaghetti

1 (1½ kg) eggplant, cut into ½-inch thick slices.

Two cups of low-sodium marinara sauce, divided

3 cups baby spinach.

1½ cup freshly grated Parmesan cheese

⅓ cup freshly chopped basil.

DIRECTIONS

1. Preheat the broiler.
2. Cook the pasta according to the package directions; drain and keep warm.
3. Meanwhile, brush both sides of the eggplant slices with cooking spray. Place eggplant in a broiler-safe 13- by 9-inch baking dish (see Note); broil for 2 minutes per side, or until just soft and lightly browned.
4. Spoon the sauce over the eggplant and top with the spinach and cheese. Return the dish to the oven and broil for 1 to 2 minutes, until thoroughly heated and the cheese has melted. Serve eggplant over pasta and garnish with basil.

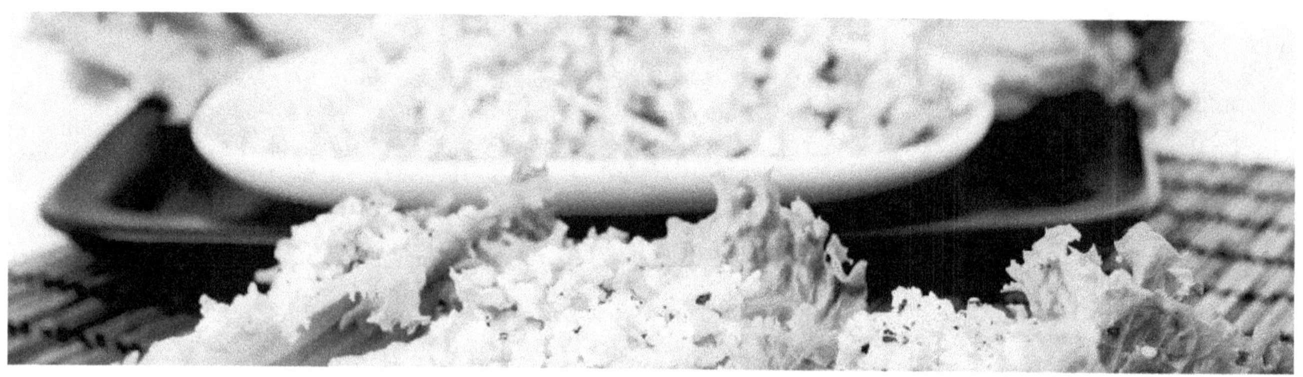

Tuna Salad with Lettuce Wraps

CALORIES: 314   **FAT: 24G**   **PROTEIN: 19G**   **CARB: 8.9G**

SERVINGS: 2   **PREP TIME: 25 MINS**   **TOTAL TIME: 25 MINS**

INGREDIENTS

Two 5 ounces. Cans high-quality canned tuna (see notes)

1/4 cup mayonnaise.

1 tsp. Dijon mustard

2 tablespoons fresh lemon juice, divided (see notes)

1/2 tsp. Celery Seed

Add salt or Vege-Sal to taste.

2 tablespoons dill pickle relish.

2 T capers.

1/4 cup thinly sliced green onions (more or less as desired)

8 big Romaine lettuce leaves were washed and dried (see notes).

1 cup of diced cherry tomatoes (optional).

One large avocado, cut small (optional)

DIRECTIONS

1. Place the tuna in a fine-mesh strainer in the sink and allow to drain thoroughly.
2. While the tuna drains, mix together the mayonnaise, Dijon mustard, lemon juice (or lime juice), celery seed, and Vege-Sal or salt.
3. Chop the tomatoes and avocados, and slice the green onions.
4. Combine the avocado with a tablespoon of lemon (or lime) juice, then toss in the tomatoes.
5. After the tuna has drained, transfer it to a bowl (with a snap-tight lid if you won't be eating it all at once).
6. Mix the dressing into the tuna first, making sure it is well distributed. Then whisk in dill pickle relish.
7. capers, and sliced green onion.
8. Separate the lettuce head and take out 8 big leaves. (I used two heads of romaine, saving the smaller inner leaves for salad greens.)
9. Wash the lettuce and spin dry in a salad spinner, or dry with paper towels if necessary.
10. Fill lettuce leaves with two heaping tablespoons of tuna mixture, top with the cherry tomato and avocado mixture, and consume with your hands.

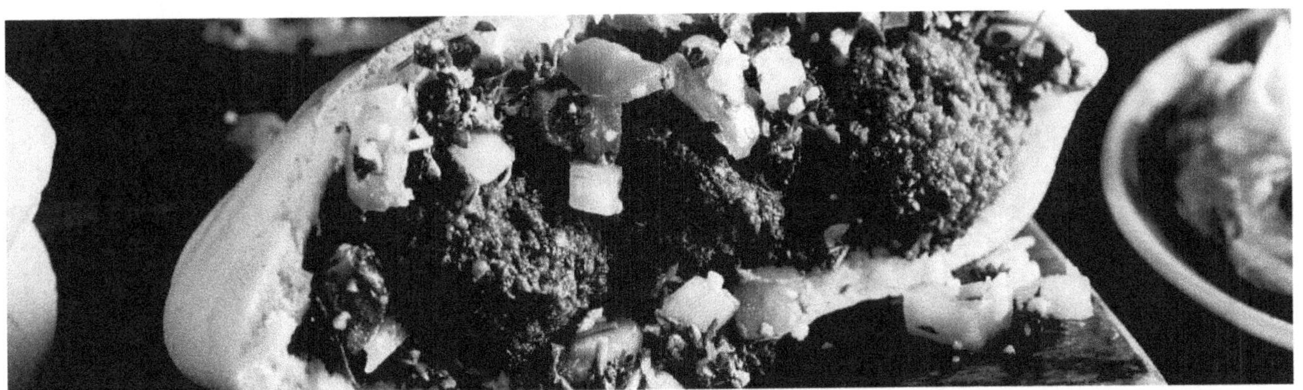

Falafel Pita Sandwich With Tahini Sauce

CALORIES: 244   **FAT: 7G**   **PROTEIN: 11G**   **CARB: 36G**

SERVINGS: 6   **PREP TIME: 30 MINS**   **TOTAL TIME: 30 MINS**

INGREDIENTS

1 15-oz BPA-free can of unsalted chickpeas (drained and rinsed).
1/4 yellow onion, chopped into three or four slices.
1/4 cup whole wheat pastry flour.
2 tablespoons fresh flat-leaved parsley
4 cloves of garlic, divided (NOTE: leave 2 cloves intact and mince 2 cloves)
1 tsp sodium-free baking powder.
1/2 teaspoon ground cumin (try Simply Organic Ground Cumin)
1/2 teaspoon of ground coriander (TRY: Simply Organic Coriander)
1/2 teaspoon sea salt.
Olive oil cooking spray
1/4 cup tahini paste.
2 tablespoons fresh lemon juice
1/4 teaspoon paprika (TRY: Simply Organic Paprika).
Six 6-inch whole-wheat pitas.
1 head green or red leaf lettuce, coarsely shredded.
1 tomato sliced into tiny wedges.
1/2 cucumber, peeled and sliced.
One low-sodium dill pickle, sliced
1/4 small red onion, thinly sliced
Harissa or other hot sauce, optional

DIRECTIONS

1. In a food processor, combine chickpeas, yellow onion, flour, parsley, whole garlic, baking powder, cumin, coriander, and salt, and pulse to make a gritty mixture, scraping down the bowl as needed. Shape the paste into 12 golf ball-sized circles and arrange them on a platter.

2. Coat a large nonstick skillet with cooking spray and heat on medium-low. To prevent crowding the skillet, work in batches and flatten the balls to about ½ inch thick using a spatula. Cook until the bottom is browned, about 4 to 5 minutes. Flip and brown the second side for 4 to 5 minutes.

3. In a separate bowl, mix together tahini, ¼ cup water, lemon juice, remaining minced garlic, and paprika.

4. Cut approximately an inch from the top of each pita to form a pocket. Fill each pita with 2 falafel and distribute lettuce, tomato, cucumber, pickle, red onion, and tahini sauce evenly. Drizzle each with harissa (if desired).

62

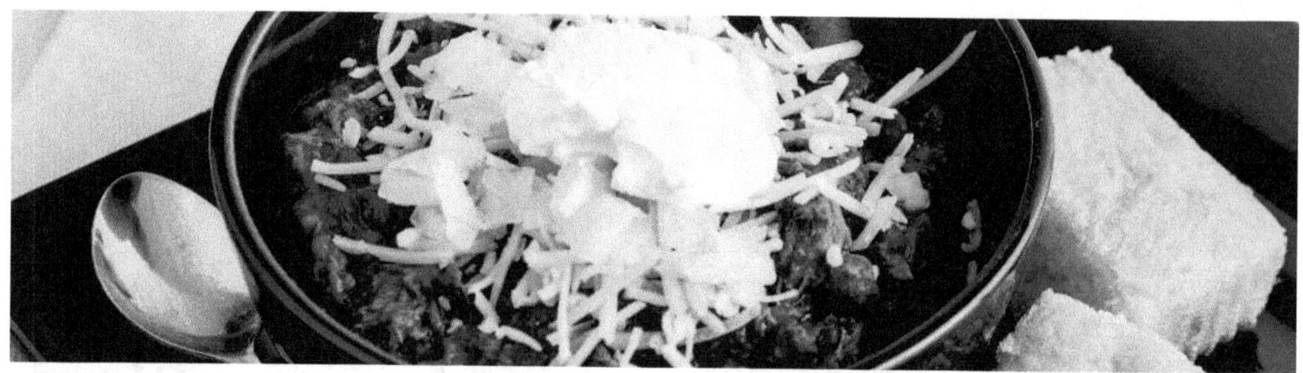

Bean and vegetable chili with cornbread

CALORIES: 429   **FAT: 14G**   **PROTEIN: 10G**   **CARB: 62G**

SERVINGS: 6   **PREP TIME: 15 MINS**   **COOK TIME: 45 MINS**

INGREDIENTS

For the Black Bean Chili
1/2 yellow onion, chopped.
One green bell pepper, chopped
3 garlic cloves, minced
2 tablespoons of olive oil.
1 tablespoon of mild chili powder.
1 teaspoon cumin.
1 teaspoon of dried oregano.
2 minced chipotle chiles in adobo + 1 tablespoon adobo sauce
Two (15-ounce) cans of black beans, drained and rinsed
1 (15 oz) can fire-roasted tomatoes.
1 1/2 cups chicken or veggie broth
2 tbsp cornflour (to thicken, optional)
Juice of 1/2 lime
Salt to taste.
Chop cilantro for serving.
For the cornmeal biscuits.
3/4 cup milk.
Juice of 1/2 lime
1 cup all-purpose flour.
3/4 cup yellow cornmeal.
1 tablespoon baking powder.
1/2 teaspoon salt.
5 tablespoons chilled vegan or dairy butter, cubed
2 tablespoons of honey.

DIRECTIONS

1. Preheat the oven to 350° F and set to convection.
2. Heat the oil in a large skillet over medium heat. Add the onion and simmer for 5-7 minutes, or until softened. Combine the green pepper, garlic, and seasonings. Cook for another 2-3 minutes, until fragrant.
3. Combine the minced chipotle peppers, adobo sauce, black beans, fire-roasted tomatoes, broth, and lime juice. Season with salt to taste.
4. To make a thicker chili, dilute the corn flour with 3 tbsp water in a separate bowl before adding to the saucepan.
5. Bring to a boil, then reduce to a low heat and simmer for 15 minutes, stirring regularly.
6. Meanwhile, prepare the biscuit dough. Whisk together the milk and lime juice, then put aside for 5 minutes to thicken.
7. In another large mixing basin, combine flour, cornmeal, baking powder, and salt. Use a fork to work the butter into the flour mixture until crumbly, then add the curdled milk and honey. Mix until just mixed.
8. Using a cookie scoop, sprinkle dough on top of the simmering chili. Bake for 15-20 minutes, until the biscuits are golden brown and fully cooked.
9. Serve heated, with any preferred toppings.

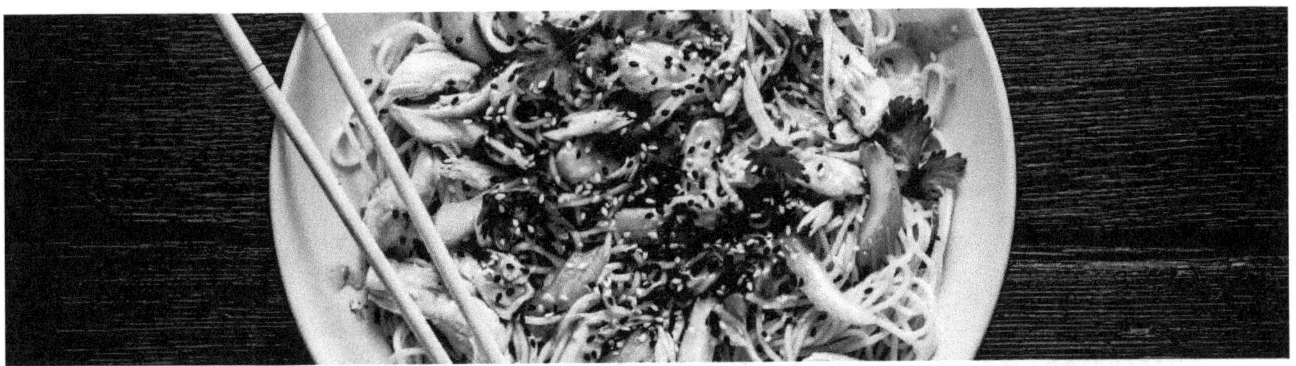

Thai Peanut Noodle Salad With Shrimp

CALORIES: 227   **FAT: 7.8G**   **PROTEIN: 14.4G**   **CARB: 26G**

SERVINGS: 12   **PREP TIME: 30 MINS**   **COOK TIME: 30 MINS**

INGREDIENTS

Salad:

8 ounces rice noodles
20 ounces cooked shrimp.
1 red pepper, diced small.
1 yellow pepper, cut small
1/2 big English cucumber, chopped.
3/4 cup shredded carrots.
3/4 cup shredded red cabbage.
1/2 small red onion, chopped
1/2 cup diced green onion
1 cup chopped cashews.
Sesame seeds.

Dressing:

1/2 cup of creamy peanut butter.
3 tablespoons of rice wine vinegar.
3 tablespoons of low-sodium soy sauce.
2 tablespoons of honey.
Juice of one lime
2 teaspoons sesame oil.
1/4 teaspoon ground ginger.
2 garlic cloves, minced
1 teaspoon sriracha.
1/2 teaspoon salt.
3-4 tbsp water to thin to the
desired consistency.

DIRECTIONS

1. Cook rice noodles, then rinse in cool water. Set aside.
2. Chop and prepare all vegetables. If fresh cooked shrimp is not used, thaw or cook it first.
3. Combine all dressing ingredients. Whisk well, then add enough water to achieve the required consistency.
4. In a large mixing bowl, combine cooked rice noodles, chopped peppers, cucumber, carrots, cabbage, red onion, green onion, half of the cashews, and shrimp.
5. Pour dressing over salad and toss with tongs until evenly coated.
6. Sprinkle with the remaining cashews and sesame seeds. Enjoy! Best served cold.

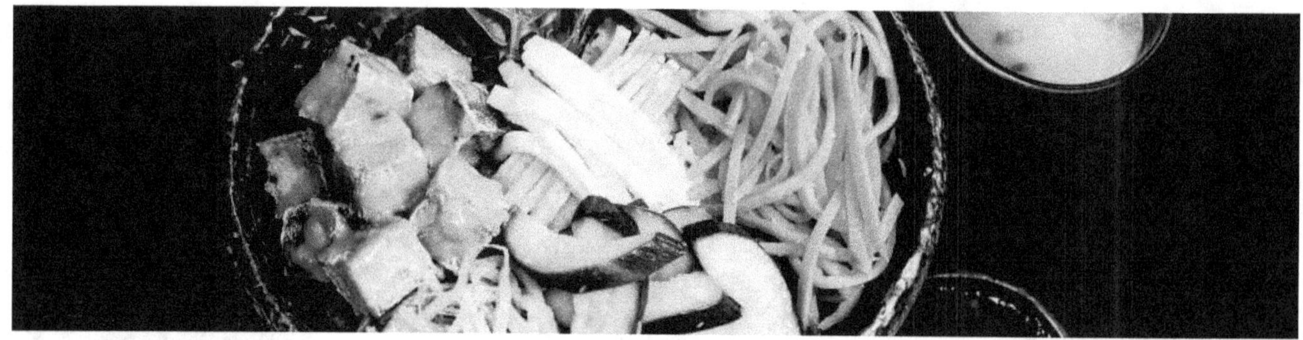

Vegetarian bibimbap with tofu and pickled vegetables

CALORIES: 595 **FAT: 19G** **PROTEIN: 22G** **CARB: 75G**

SERVINGS: 4 **PREP TIME: 20 MINS** **COOK TIME: 40 MINS**

INGREDIENTS

For the Pickled Vegetables:

1 cup daikon radish matchsticks.
One cup carrot matchsticks
1/4 teaspoon salt.
One teaspoon of sugar.
1/3 cup rice vinegar.
Add 1/3 cup warm water.

For The Tofu:

One 12 ounce container of House Foods Extra Firm Tofu, chopped into bite-sized portions
Add 2 tablespoons of soy sauce.
2 teaspoons cornstarch.
Divide 2 teaspoons of vegetable oil.
Continue ■

65

DIRECTIONS

Pickled Vegetables:

1. To make the pickled veggies, combine the daikon, carrot, salt, sugar, vinegar, and warm water in a big glass jar with a lid.

2. Shake thoroughly to dissolve the salt and sugar. Set aside for pickling (at least 10-15 minutes).

TOFU:

3. Place the sliced tofu between two double layers of paper towels. Gently massage the tofu to absorb any extra liquid.

4. To dry the tofu's outside, use a fresh paper towel. In a small bowl, mix together the soy sauce and cornstarch until well incorporated.

5. In a large nonstick pan, heat 1 tablespoon vegetable oil over medium heat.
6.........

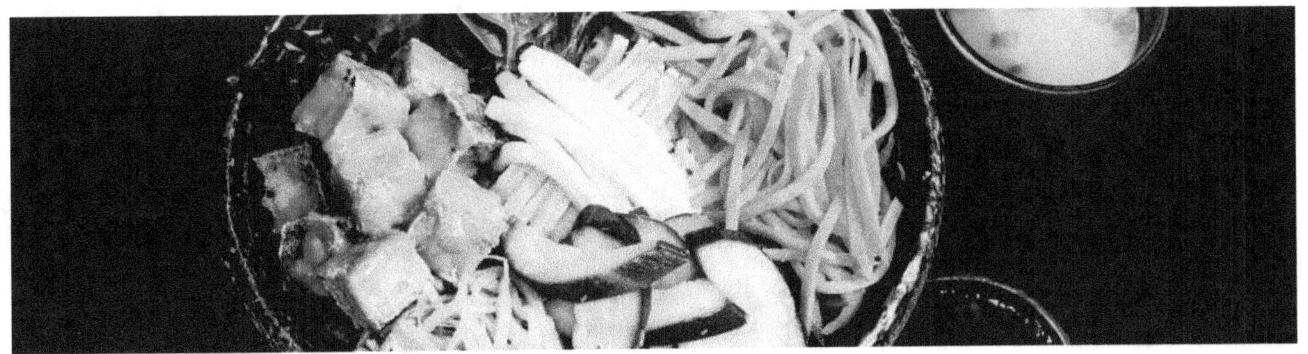

INGREDIENTS

For the cucumbers:

1 cup thinly sliced English (or other seedless) cucumber
Add 1/2 teaspoon sesame oil
1/8 teaspoon roasted sesame seeds.

For the mushrooms.

4 oz brown mushrooms, sliced
One tablespoon of vegetable oil
For the Spinach
6 cups baby spinach leaves.
Add 2 tablespoons vegetable oil.
1/2 teaspoon finely minced garlic.
Add 1/2 teaspoon sesame oil
1/8 teaspoon roasted sesame seeds.
1 finely minced scallion.

For the Bibimbap Sauce

Add 2 tablespoons gochujang.
2 teaspoons of honey.
Add 2 tablespoons of sesame oil.
Add 2 teaspoons of water.
Add 2 tablespoons of rice vinegar.
Add 1 teaspoon toasted sesame seeds.

For The Bibimbap Bowls

4 cups of Jasmine rice.
Four fried eggs.
1 cup bean sprouts.

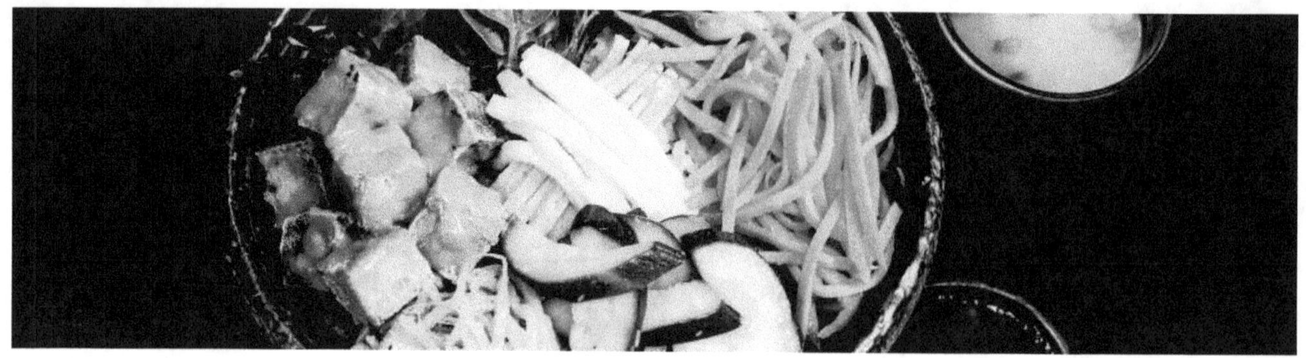

DIRECTIONS

6. Toss half of the tofu in the soy sauce and cornstarch mixture, then immediately transfer to a hot pan and cook for 1-2 minutes per side, or until golden brown. Transfer to a plate lined with paper towels to drain. Repeat with the remaining tablespoon of oil and the second half of tofu.

CUCUMBERS:

7. Use a paper towel to squeeze any extra moisture from the cucumbers. Toss the cucumbers in sesame oil and toasted sesame seeds. Set aside.

MUSHROOMS:

8. Heat the vegetable oil in a large skillet over medium-high heat. Cook the sliced mushrooms in a single layer until golden brown, about 2-3 minutes per side. Set aside.

SPINACH

9. Heat 2 teaspoons of oil in a large skillet over medium heat. Add the spinach leaves and cook for 1-2 minutes, or until wilted. Rinse the spinach immediately with cool water. Squeeze out any excess juice with your hands until the spinach feels dry.

10. Combine the spinach, minced garlic, sesame oil, sesame seeds, and scallions

BIBIMBAP SAUCE:

11. Tomake the sauce, combine the gochujang, honey, sesame oil, water, rice vinegar, and sesame seeds in a small bowl.

BIBIMBAP BOWLING:

12. Divide 1 cup rice among four separate serving bowls. Top with one-quarter of the fried tofu and one fried egg each.

13. Serve with prepared toppings (pickled vegetables, cucumber, mushrooms, spinach, bean sprouts, and sauce) and enable guests to customize their bowls.

DINNER

RECIPES

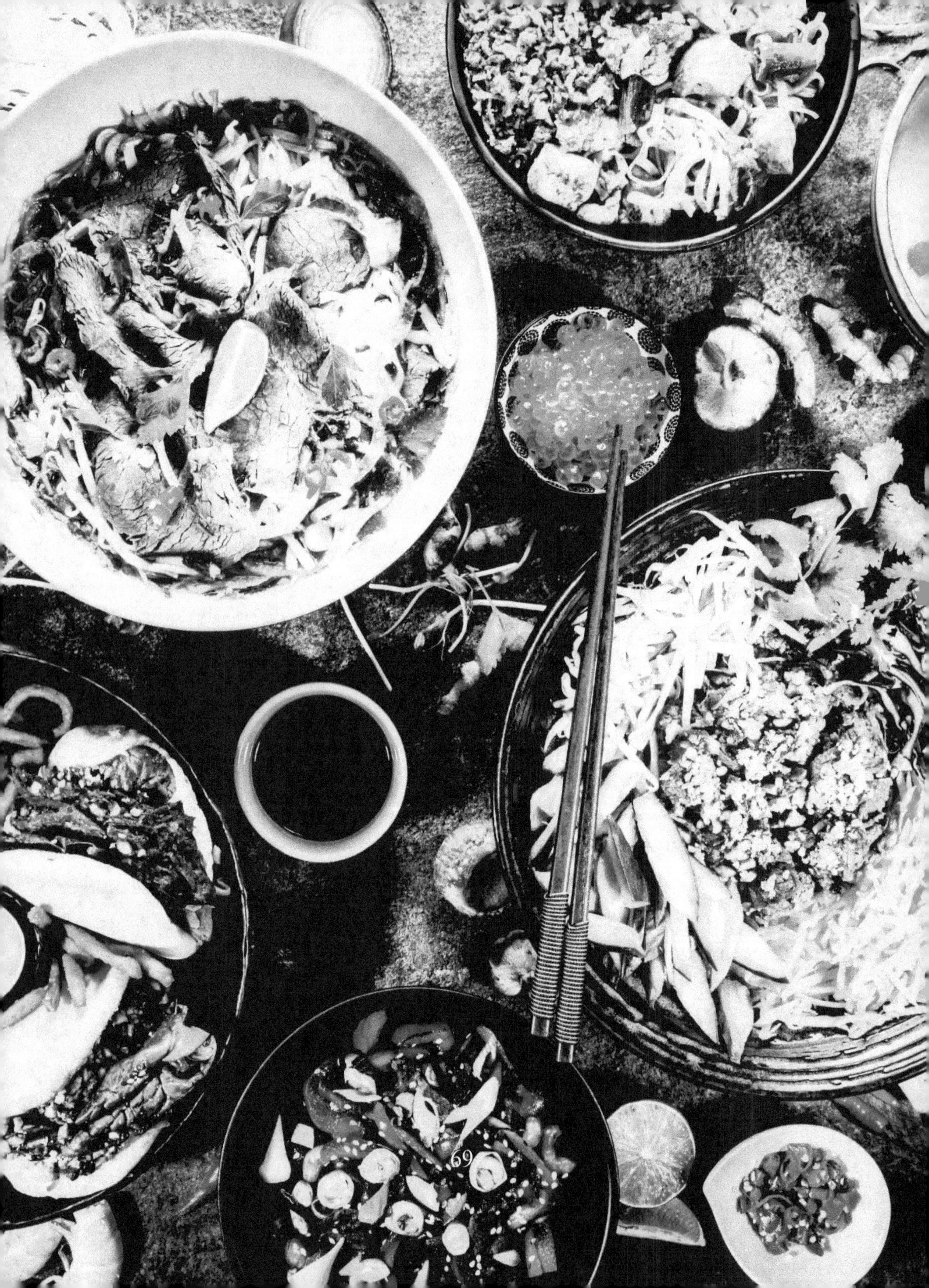

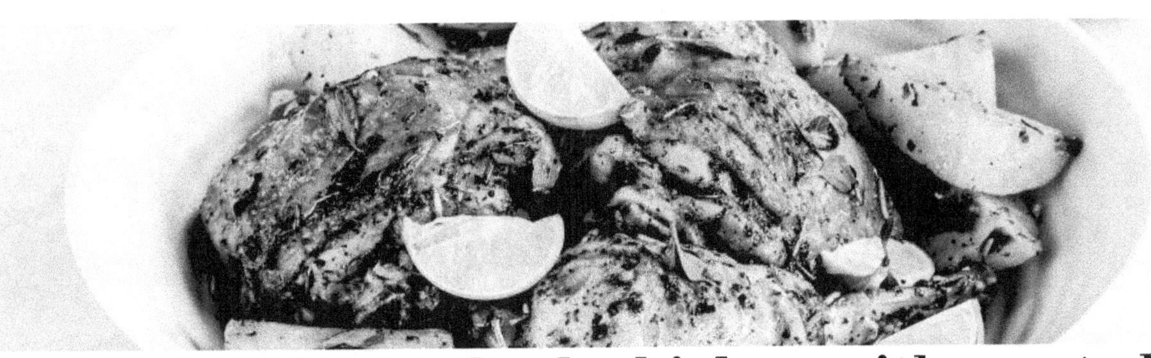

Baked lemon herb chicken with roasted vegetables.

CALORIES: 500   **FAT: 22G**   **PROTEIN: 47G**   **CARB: 25G**

SERVINGS: 4   **PREP TIME: 15 MINS**   **TOTAL TIME: 45 MINS**

INGREDIENTS

1 pound tiny red-skinned potatoes, quartered

2 medium carrots, sliced into 1 inch chunks.

Two celery stalks, peeled and chopped into 1-inch pieces.

1 medium red onion, sliced into half-inch wedges

2 teaspoons of olive oil.

Kosher salt, freshly ground black pepper.

3 bone-in, skin-on chicken breasts (about 1 3/4 pounds)

1 teaspoon of poultry seasoning.

One lemon, halved

1/4 cup chopped fresh parsley.

DIRECTIONS

1. Preheat the oven to 450 degrees Fahrenheit with the rack at the highest position. On a rimmed baking sheet, toss the potatoes, carrots, celery, and onions with 1 teaspoon olive oil, 1/2 teaspoon salt, and a few grinds of pepper. Arrange in a single layer. Roast for about 20 minutes, stirring halfway through, until the veggies are gently browned and the potatoes have just begun to soften.

2. ....

70

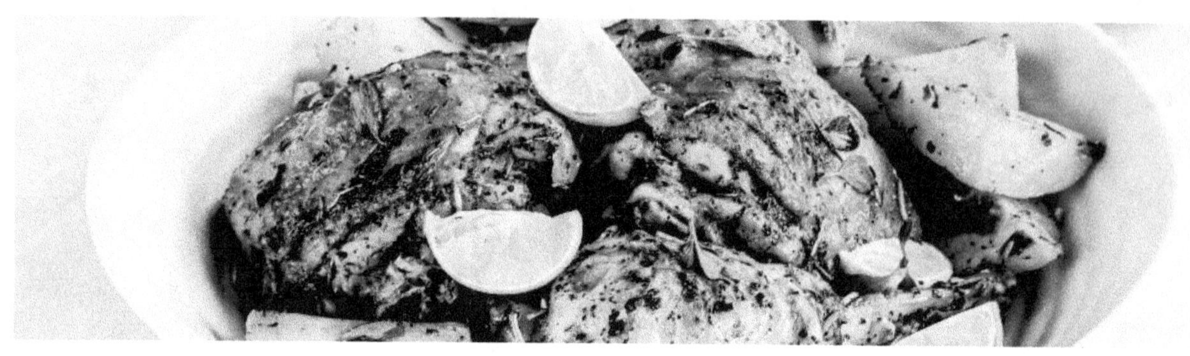

DIRECTIONS

2. Meanwhile, rub the remaining 1 teaspoon oil into the chicken breast skin and season with the poultry seasoning and 1/2 teaspoon salt. Once the veggies have softened, place the chicken breasts on top and roast for 20 to 25 minutes, or until the skin is golden brown and the chicken has reached an internal temperature of 165 degrees Fahrenheit.

3. Allow the chicken breasts to rest for a few minutes. Toss the roasted veggies with the juice from one lemon half and the parsley. Cut the bones out of the chicken breasts and slice the meat. Divide the chicken and roasted veggies onto four plates. Cut the remaining lemon half into wedges to serve alongside.

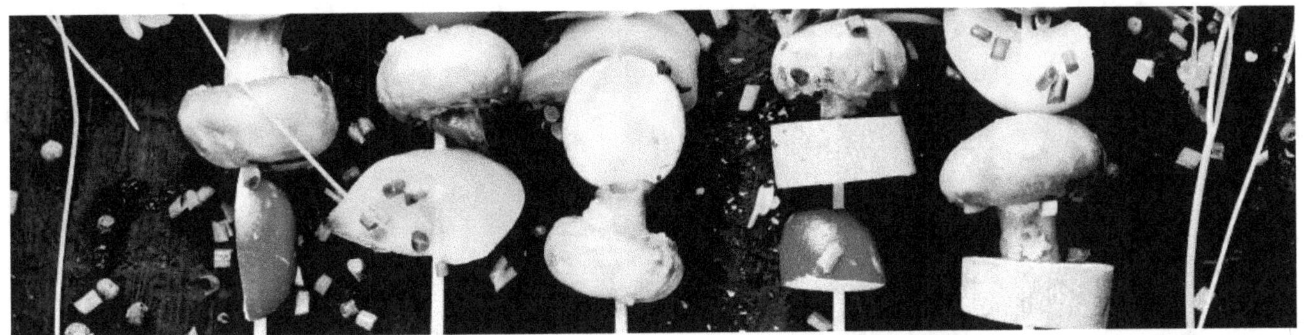

Grilled Shrimp Skewers with Vegetable Quinoa Bowl

CALORIES: 345 **FAT: 7.5G** **PROTEIN: 37.2G** **CARB: 17G**

SERVINGS: 6 **PREP TIME: 5 MINS** **TOTAL TIME: 15 MINS**

INGREDIENTS

1 pound Shrimp, deveined

1 tablespoon of olive oil.

1/2 teaspoon salt.

1/8 teaspoon black pepper.

Juice from 1/2 lemon

1/4 teaspoon paprika.

1/2 teaspoon dried oregano.

1/4 teaspoon ginger paste.

3 cups assorted vegetables (zucchini, eggplant, red and green peppers, white onion)

DIRECTIONS

1. Spices: In a small bowl, combine salt, black pepper, paprika, and dried oregano.

2. Marinate the Shrimp: Place the shrimp in a bowl, drizzle with olive oil and lemon juice, and season with seasonings. Toss to coat. Cover and let marinate for about 30 minutes (or overnight).

3. Soak the Stick: If using disposable wooden skewers, soak them in water for an hour before using. Alternatively, wrap the last 3-inch end with aluminum foil.

4. Thread the shrimp onto the skewers, alternately with the vegetables.

5. Preheat the grill to 350°F, then cook the shrimp and vegetables for 8-10 minutes (more or less). Brush each side with olive oil after flipping it to cook the other side.

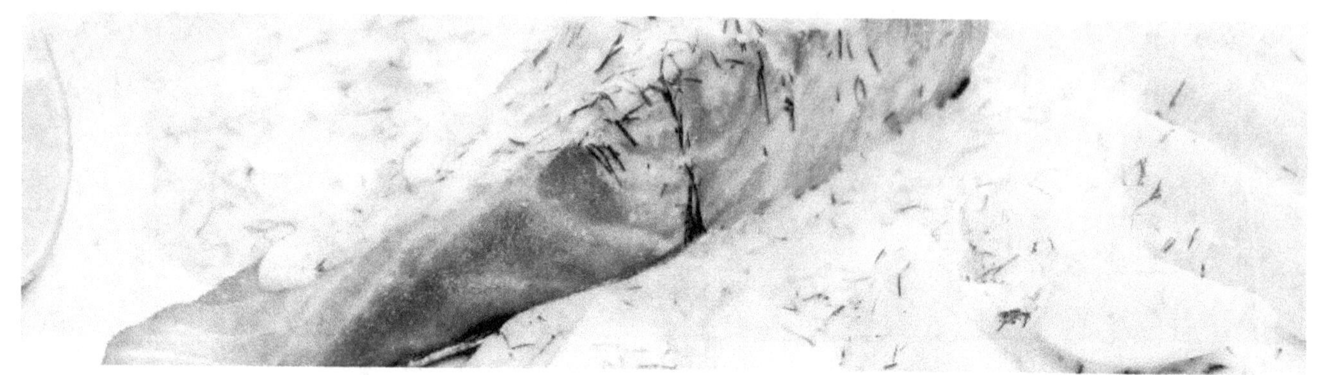

Baked Salmon with Lemon Dill Sauce

CALORIES: 334   **FAT: 20G**   **PROTEIN: 36G**   **CARB: 2G**

SERVINGS: 1   **PREP TIME: 10 MINS**   **TOTAL TIME: 20 MINS**

INGREDIENTS

4 6 oz salmon fillets (we prefer Costco salmon)

1 tablespoon of olive oil.

Add salt and pepper to taste.

Lemon wedges for garnish, if desired.

Lemon Dill Sauce

1/3 cup Greek yogurt.

2 tablespoons mayonnaise.

1.5 tbsp dill (chopped if using fresh) (we use freeze dried, but fresh also works great).

2 tablespoons lemon juice.

1 teaspoon lemon zest.

1 teaspoon granulated garlic.

Salt & pepper, to taste.

DIRECTIONS

1. Preheat the oven to 400 degrees Fahrenheit.
2. Place the fish on a foil-lined baking tray. Drizzle the top with olive oil, salt, and pepper. Bake 12-16 minutes, depending on the thickness of the salmon filet. When the internal temperature reaches 135 degrees, remove from the oven and allow to rest until 145 degrees (the safe cooking temperature for salmon).
3. While the fish is baking, combine the dill sauce ingredients. Set aside.
4. When the salmon is cooked to your liking, spread dill sauce on top. If preferred, garnish with a lemon wedge. Serve.

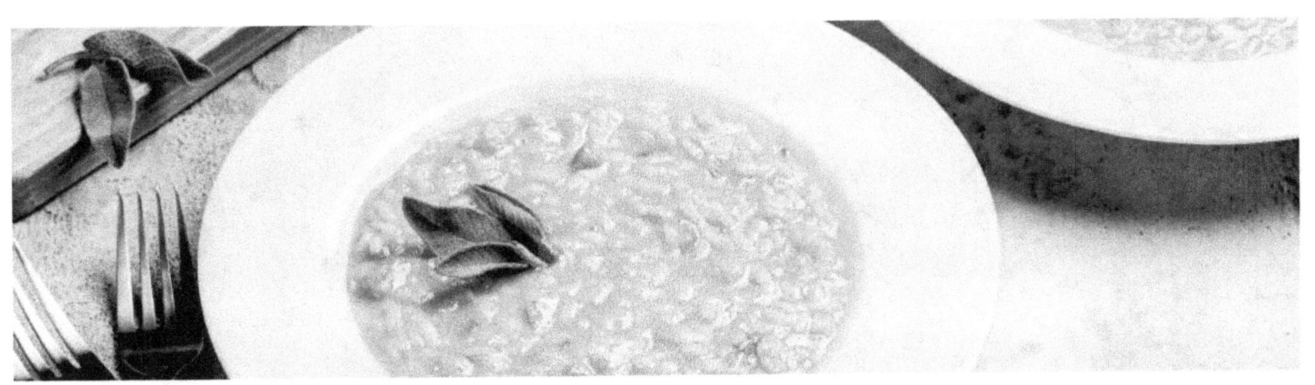

Pumpkin & Sage Risotto

CALORIES: 345   **FAT: 17G**   **PROTEIN: 11G**   **CARB: 38G**

SERVINGS: 3   **PREP TIME: 25 MINS**   **TOTAL TIME: 23 MINS**

INGREDIENTS

For the Pumpkin Risotto
570ml (1 pint) vegetable or chicken stock
1 small onion, chopped.
12 fresh sage leaves, freshly chopped
2 tablespoons olive oil.
170g/6oz Arborio rice
250g/9oz pumpkin or butternut squash,
chopped tiny.
50g/2oz butter
salt, freshly ground black pepper.
For crispy sage
12–16 fresh sage leaves
2 tablespoons sunflower oil.

To garnish.

A piece of fresh Parmesan or vegetarian
Parmesan-style grated cheese (optional)

DIRECTIONS

1. Heat the stock until almost boiling, then reduce to a very low heat. In a separate heavy-bottomed skillet, cook the onion in oil over low heat until tender but not browned. Cook for a few minutes more after adding the chopped sage.

2. Add the rice and stir for a few seconds to coat the grains with oil, then pour in one-third of the stock and bring to a medium simmer.

3. Cook until nearly all of the stock is absorbed. Add the pumpkin or squash and a bit more stock, then boil gently until the stock is absorbed.

4. ......

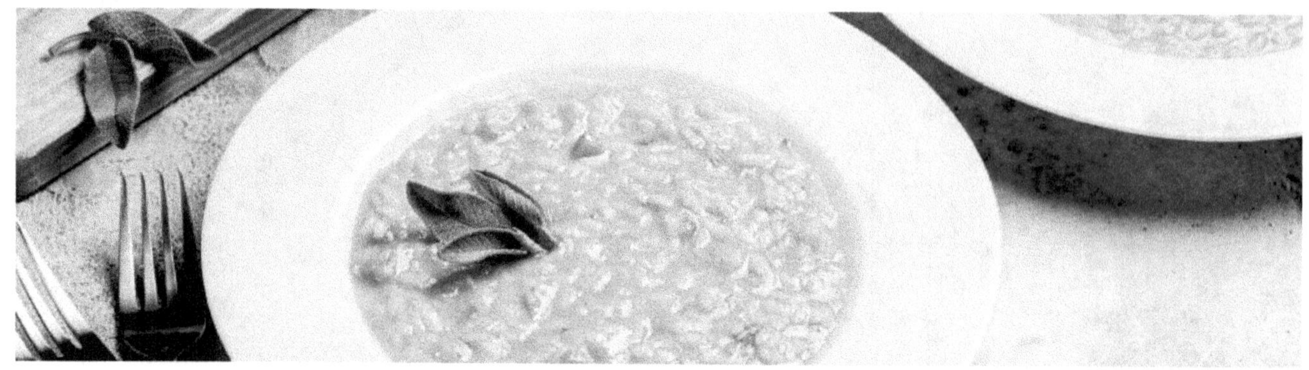

DIRECTIONS

4. From there, add more stock a little at a time, until the pumpkin is mushy and the rice is al dente (with a slight bite). You may not need all of the stock, but the consistency should be loose and creamy.

5. When the risotto is almost done, heat the sunflower oil in a small skillet and quickly fry the sage leaves until crispy, which takes only a few seconds.

6. Add the butter to the risotto and season with salt and pepper. Divide evenly among four bowls and top with a few crispy sage leaves. Bring cheese and a grater to the table so your guests may serve themselves.

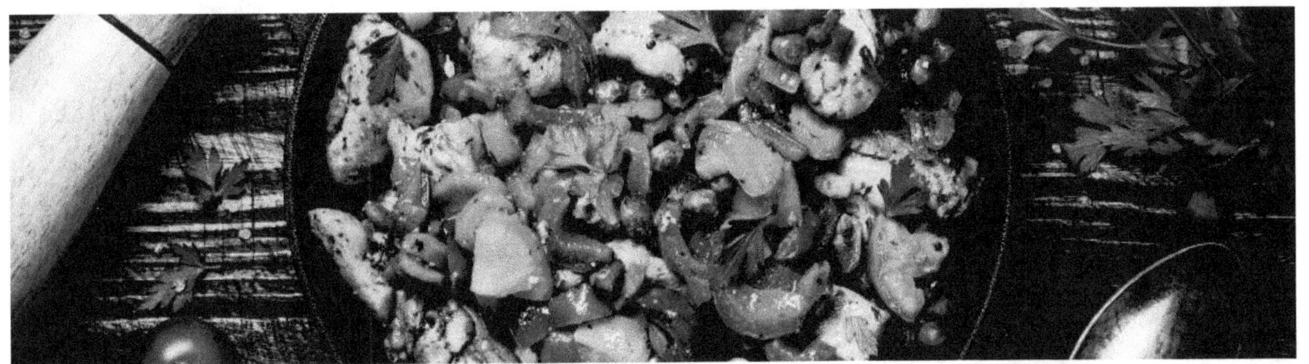

Shrimp and Vegetable Stir-Fry

CALORIES: 317   **FAT: 6G**   **PROTEIN: 24G**   **CARB: 47G**

SERVINGS: 6   **PREP TIME: 20 MINS**   **COOK TIME: 15 MINS**

INGREDIENTS

Two cups instant brown rice
One ¾ cups water
Six tablespoons soy sauce
¼ cup honey
Six tablespoons of water
Two tablespoons of cornstarch
2 tablespoons of cider vinegar
Two tablespoons of olive oil
Two cloves garlic, chopped
Two cups broccoli florets
One cup baby carrots
One small white onion, chopped
½ teaspoon black pepper
1 cup sliced fresh mushrooms
1 ½ pounds uncooked medium
shrimp, peeled and deveined

DIRECTIONS

1. In a microwave-safe bowl, combine rice and water. Cover and microwave on high for 8 minutes, or until the water has been completely absorbed. Fluff with a fork, then cover and set aside.
2. In a small mixing dish, combine soy sauce, water, honey, cider vinegar, and cornstarch. Set aside.
3. In a nonstick skillet, heat the olive oil on medium heat. Stir in the garlic and heat for 10 seconds more.
4. Cook and mix in the broccoli, carrots, onion, and black pepper for approximately 5 minutes, or until the vegetables are soft. Stir in the mushrooms and simmer for another 2 minutes. Remove the vegetables from the skillet and set them aside.

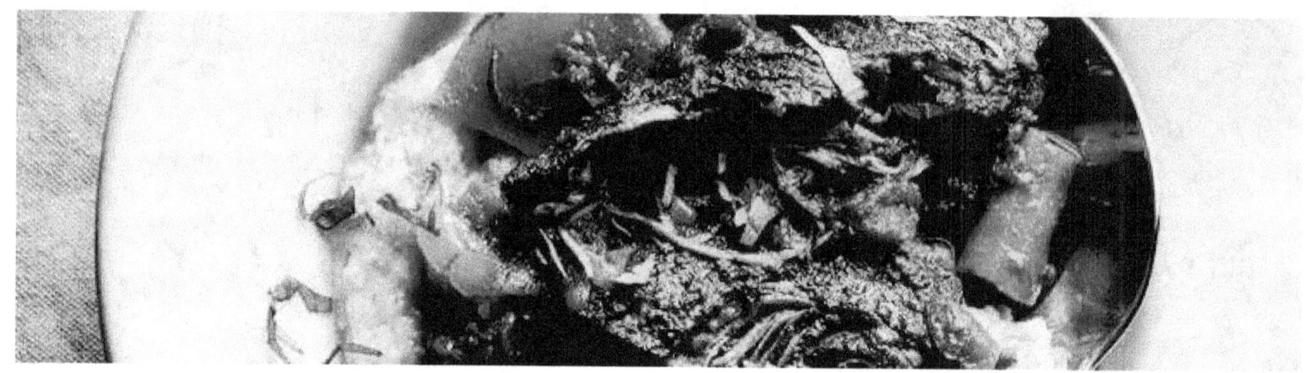

Sesame Ginger Beef and Broccoli Stir-Fry

SERVINGS: 3   **PREP TIME: 30 MINS**   **TOTAL TIME: 30 MINS**

INGREDIENTS

The basics:

1 lb. beef flank steak, thinly sliced
1 head broccoli, chopped into florets
2 tablespoons of vegetable oil.
3 garlic cloves, thinly cut or minced.
One 1-inch knob of freshly peeled ginger, grated or sliced
1.5 cups of uncooked white rice or brown rice (or one package of cauliflower rice)
thinly sliced green onions for serving.

The Sauce:

1/4 cup low-sodium soy sauce
1/4 cup water.
1/3 cup brown sugar (substitute coconut sugar).
1 tablespoon of sambal oelek.
1 tablespoon rice vinegar (substitute for white vinegar).
1 tablespoon of sesame oil.
1 tablespoon of cornstarch.

DIRECTIONS

1. Beef Preparation: Freeze the beef for 30 minutes to an hour to make it easier to slice. Thinly slice against the grain. Toss the beef strips with a hefty pinch of coarse salt and set them to rest while you prepare the remaining ingredients. (All of this is optional, but highly recommended for flavor and texture.)
2. Whisk the sauce ingredients together.
3. Rice: Cook the rice according to the package directions.
4. Stir Fry Time: Preheat a big, heavy skillet over medium heat. Add a swirl of oil. Working in batches, arrange the beef in a single layer. Allow it to rest undisturbed for a minute or two to obtain a beautiful browning of the meat. Cook each slice until browned and delicious. Remove beef from the pan.
5. Broccoli: Add a splash of oil to the same pan. Add the broccoli and stir fry for 2-3 minutes, or until bright green. (I occasionally add a dash of water to steam it a little.) Remove broccoli from the pan.
6. .....

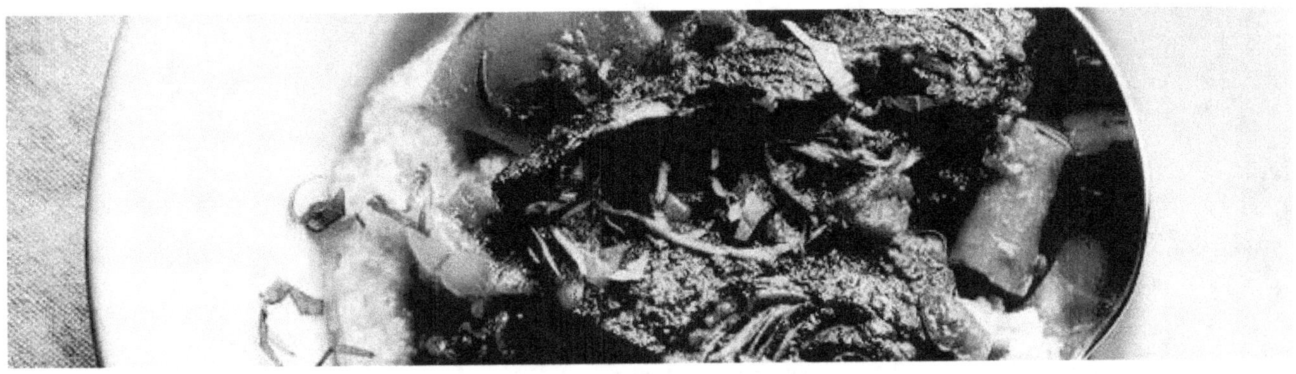

DIRECTIONS

6. Finally, reduce the heat and allow the pan to cool somewhat. Add one final swish of oil. Sauté the ginger and garlic for 1–2 minutes. Add the sauce and stir until it thickens and becomes sticky. Add the beef and broccoli back in. Toss lightly to coat.

7. Yummy! Serve with rice, thinly sliced green onions, and sesame seeds.

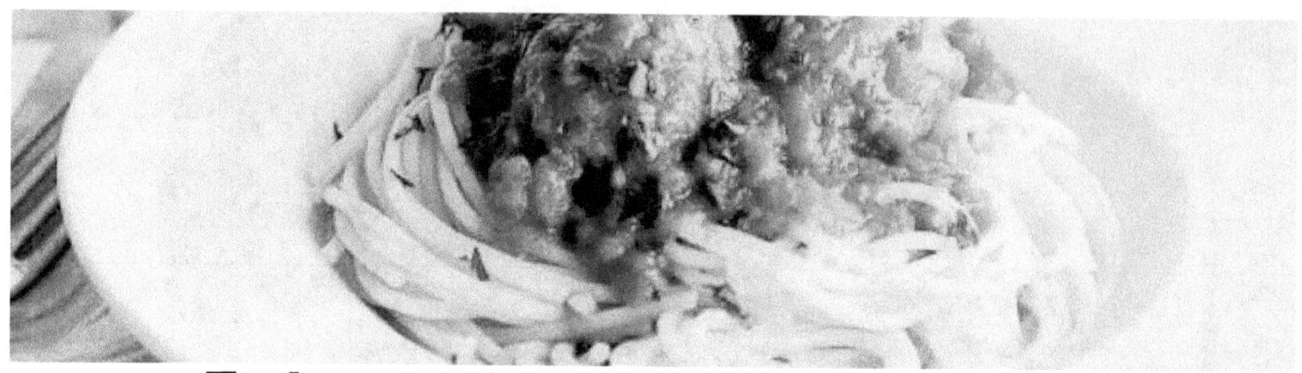

Turkey meatballs with marinara sauce and whole wheat spaghetti

CALORIES: 489   **FAT: 2.5G**   **PROTEIN: 36G**   **CARB: 87G**

SERVINGS: 6   **PREP TIME: 25 MINS**   **TOTAL TIME: 35 MINS**

INGREDIENTS

Marinara Sauce

14 oz. tinned, no-salt-added, or low-sodium sliced carrots.
14.4 oz. Packed and frozen pepper stir-fry (onions and peppers) (thawed)
1 medium zucchini, chopped.
4 cloves fresh garlic, minced

OR

2 tsp. jarred, minced garlic
52 oz. Cubed, salt-free, or low-sodium tomato (crushed)
2 tsp. Salt-free, dried Italian spice blend

Whole wheat spaghetti with turkey meatballs.
1 lb. Extra-lean or fat-free ground turkey breast (95-99% lean)
1/4 tsp. Black Pepper
1/2 cup whole grain cereal flakes (crushed is optional)
1 lb. Whole wheat pasta

DIRECTIONS

Marinara Sauce

1. Add carrots to a big pot (not yet heated). Mash with a fork or potato masher. Add the stir-fry vegetables, zucchini, garlic, smashed tomatoes, and spice mixture.
2. Bring to a boil on high heat. Cover and decrease the heat to medium-low until the sauce is simmering.

Whole wheat spaghetti with turkey meatballs

3. In a bowl, combine the turkey, pepper, cereal, and parsley. Form the meat mixture into golf-sized meatballs, about 20 to 25 in total.
4. Add the meatballs to the simmering sauce, being sure to cover the bulk of them with sauce. Cover and cook for 20 to 25 minutes, or until the meatballs are thoroughly cooked.
5. Make spaghetti according to the package directions (without the salt and fat). Serve with marinara a
nd meatballs.

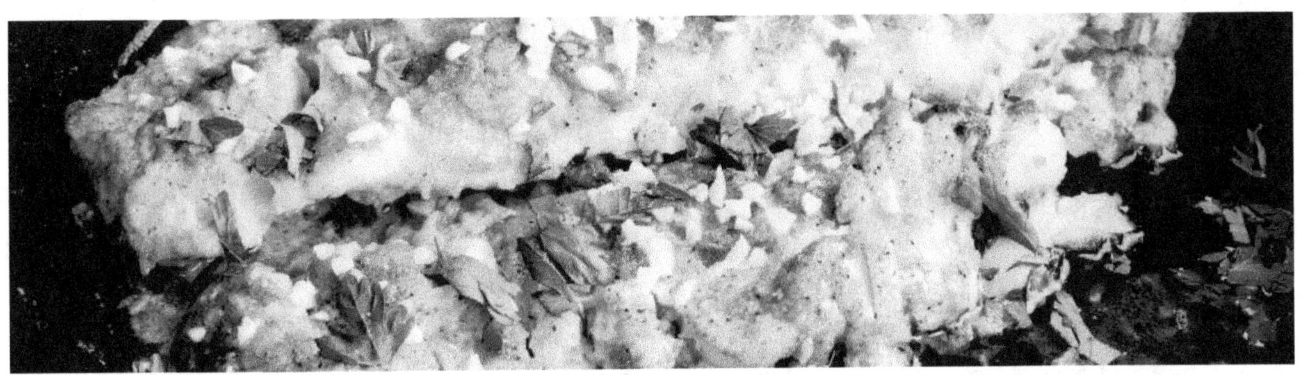

Lemon-garlic Baked Cod with Quinoa

CALORIES: 555   **FAT: 32G**   **PROTEIN: 31.9G**   **CARB: 32G**

SERVINGS: 4   **PREP TIME: 20 MINS**   **TOTAL TIME: 30 MINS**

INGREDIENTS

1 1/2 cups water.

1/2 teaspoon of fine salt, divided.

1 cup (6 1/2 ounces) uncooked quinoa (ideally multicolored)

Four skinless cod filets (1 1/2 inch thick, 5 to 6 ounces each), thawed if frozen

2 teaspoons cornstarch

1/4 teaspoon of freshly ground black pepper.

1 lemon.

1/2 cup extra virgin olive oil.

3 garlic cloves, chopped or grated.

A pinch of sweet paprika.

A pinch of cayenne pepper (optional).

DIRECTIONS

1. Preheat the oven to 400 degrees with a rack in the center.
2. In a medium saucepan over high heat, bring 1 1/2 cups water and 1/4 teaspoon salt to a boil. Reduce the heat to low, cover, and cook for 15 minutes, or until the water has been absorbed and the quinoa is cooked. (If the quinoa is still wet, uncover, reduce the heat to medium-low, and cook for another minute, stirring occasionally.) Remove from the heat and cover.
3. While the quinoa cooks, pat the cod dry and season with the cornstarch, remaining salt, and black pepper.
4. Slice the lemon in half. Juice half and cut the other half into four wedges.

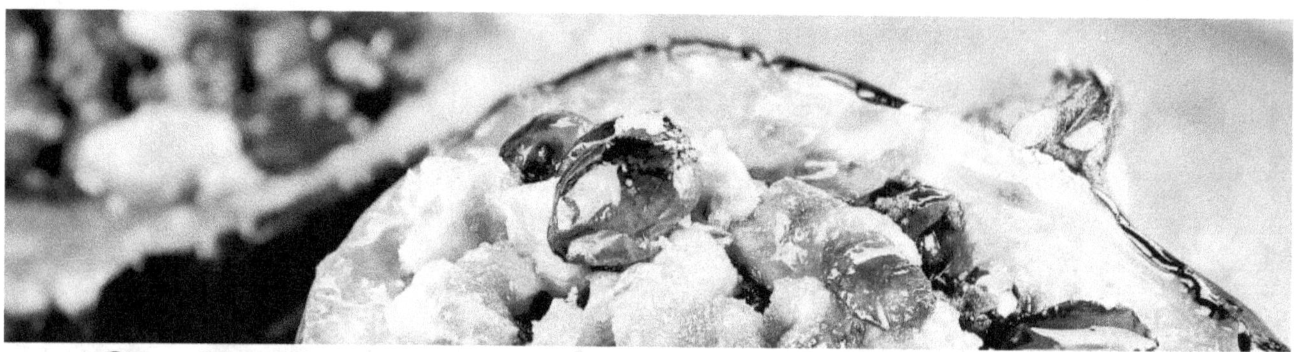

Stuffed acorn squash with wild rice and cranberries

CALORIES: 15   **FAT: 1G**   **PROTEIN: 4G**   **CARB: 26G**

SERVINGS: 4   **PREP TIME: 15 MINS**   **COOK TIME: 45 MINS**

INGREDIENTS

Two medium-sized acorn squash.

3-4 teaspoons of refined coconut oil for sautéing.

8 oz. sliced mushrooms (white, bella, or cremini)

1 tiny yellow onion, chopped.

Two celery stalks, chopped

2 cups vegetable broth (I use low sodium)

1 and ¼ cups wild rice blend, uncooked

⅓ cup dried cranberries.

¼ cup chopped walnuts.

SEASONINGS

½ teaspoon dried basil.

½ teaspoon dried thyme.

⅓ teaspoon dry parsley.

⅓ teaspoon garlic powder.

Himalayan pink salt, to taste*

Pepper to taste.

DIRECTIONS

ACORN SQUASH

1. Begin by preheating your oven to 425°F and lining a baking sheet with parchment.

2. Now lay the squash on its side. Carefully remove the bottom point and trim the stem so that it may lie level on both sides. (For more information, refer to the post above.)

3. While the squash is on its side, use a sharp knife to cut horizontally through the center to create two flower-shaped halves. A sharp knife is essential for this task, as it may require some effort. If you're having difficulty cutting through it, rock the knife back and forth to assist it slide through.

4. Remove the seeds and pulp with a spoon or ice cream scoop. Discard them or keep them to roast.

5. Brush/rub coconut oil on the squash's top and inside. Then place them cut side down on the baking pan.

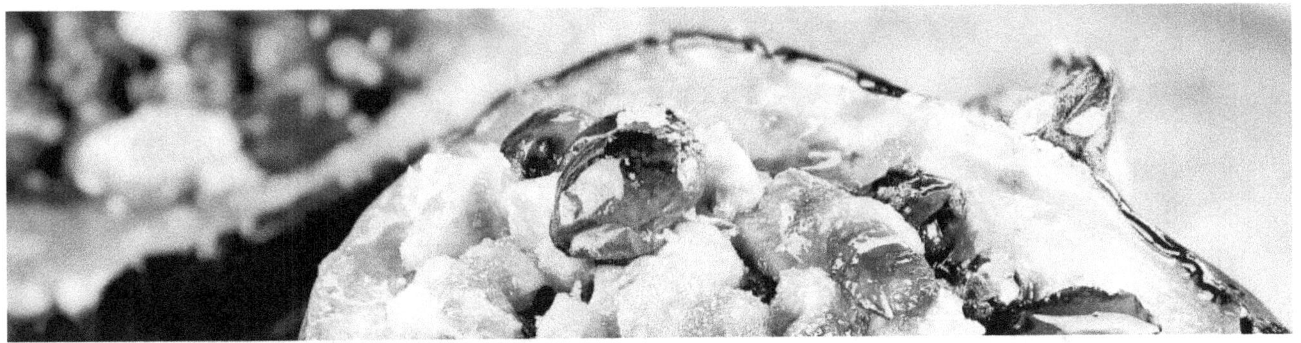

DIRECTIONS

6. Put the baking sheet in the oven on the center rack. Roast the squash at 425°F for 30-40 minutes, or until a fork can easily pierce the center.

7. Remove the squash from the oven and let it cool on the baking sheet for 15 minutes before handling.

Wild Rice With Mushrooms

8. While the acorn squash are baking, prepare the wild rice and mushroom filling.

9. Sauté the onion and celery in a pot with a little oil until they change color and texture. Approximately 5 minutes.

10. Add the broth, wild rice, and seasoning to the pot. Cover and heat to a boil. Once boiling, reduce the heat and simmer for 40-45 minutes, or until the rice is completely cooked. If the rice is still firm after cooking, add 1-2 tablespoons of liquid and cook for a little longer.

11. While the rice is cooking, heat a little oil in a skillet and sauté the mushrooms until soft. Approximately 10-15 minutes.

12. Combine the mushrooms, cranberries, and walnuts in the pot with the thoroughly cooked wild rice.

Stuffing the Acorn Squash.

13. Once the squash has cooled enough to handle, flip them over. Leave them on the baking sheet and ladle the wild rice mixture into the hollows of each squash half.

14. Place them back in the oven and bake for another 8-10 minutes.

15. Serve as is, or garnish with fresh parsley or thyme.

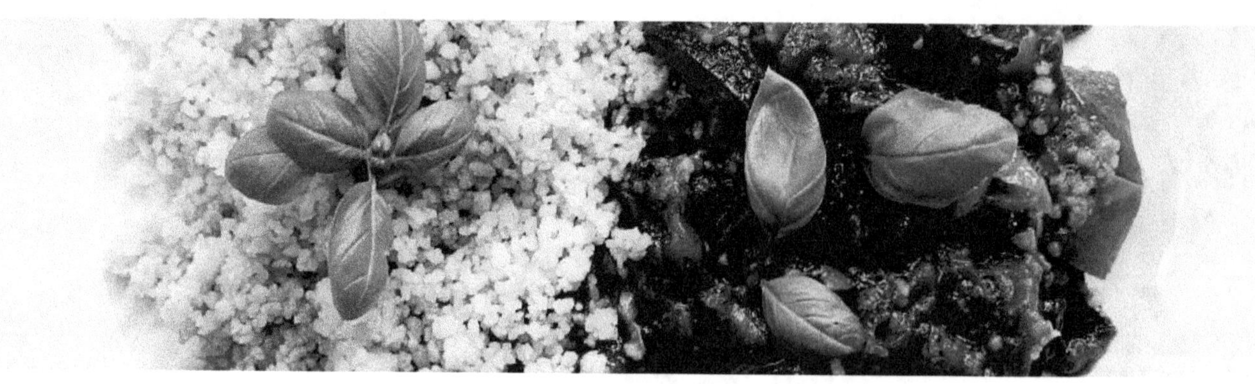

Ratatouille with Couscous

CALORIES: 235   **FAT: 1.7G**   **PROTEIN: 5.4G**   **CARB: 32.8G**

SERVINGS: 6   **PREP TIME: 10 MINS**   **COOK TIME: 20 MINS**

INGREDIENTS

For Roasted Ratatouille:

½ huge globe eggplant.
2 small to medium zucchinis
Two red bell peppers.
2 cups cherry tomatoes.
Half of a huge red onion.
4 huge cloves of garlic in their skin.
3 teaspoons dried oregano, basil, or thyme
Salt and pepper.
1/4 cup olive oil.

For Couscous:

1 tablespoon of olive oil.
1.5 cups dry pearl couscous (also called Israeli couscous)
2.25 cups water.
½ teaspoon of kosher salt.
½ cup fresh parsley for garnish.

DIRECTIONS

1. To make Roasted Ratatouille, begin by preparing your vegetables. Cut eggplant into ½ inch cubes and place in a colander in the sink. Salt heavily and set aside for 5 minutes (this will extract some bitterness). Rinse the salt off and set aside. Preheat the oven to 400 degrees Fahrenheit.

2. Wash all produce and chop the zucchini, peppers, cherry tomatoes, and red onion into similarly small pieces. Spread everything (including your reserved eggplant) out on two lined baking pans, forming an even layer as possible. Add four garlic cloves (in peel) to the sheet. Sprinkle dry herbs, salt, and pepper liberally across both sheets. Spread olive oil over both and stir to coat.

3. ....

83

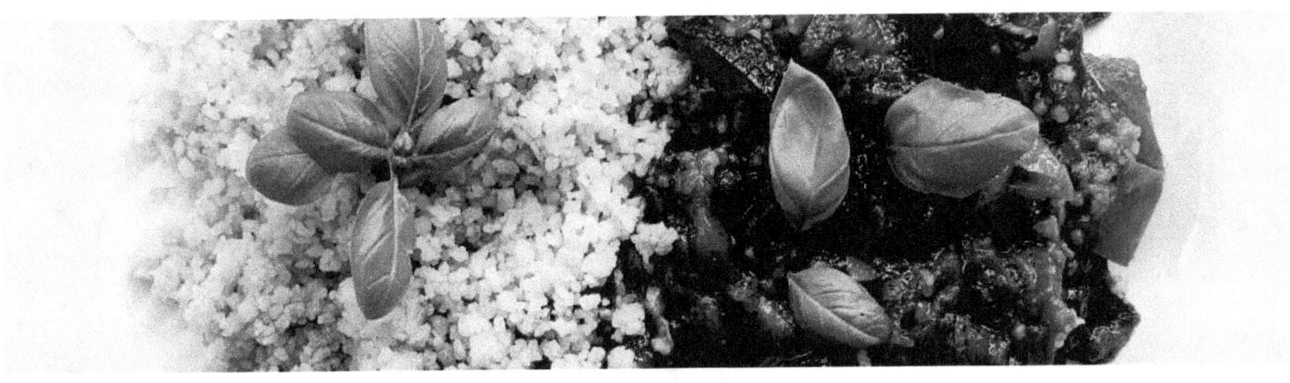

DIRECTIONS

4. To make Roasted Ratatouille, begin by preparing your vegetables. Cut eggplant into ½ inch cubes and place in a colander in the sink. Salt heavily and set aside for 5 minutes (this will extract some bitterness). Rinse the salt off and set aside. Preheat the oven to 400 degrees Fahrenheit.

5. Wash all produce and chop the zucchini, peppers, cherry tomatoes, and red onion into similarly small pieces. Spread everything (including your reserved eggplant) out on two lined baking pans, forming an even layer as possible. Add four garlic cloves (in peel) to the sheet. Sprinkle dry herbs, salt, and pepper liberally across both sheets. Spread olive oil over both and stir to coat.

6. Roast the vegetables for 20 minutes, until they are equally golden brown. Keep an eye out for any symptoms of burning. While the vegetables are roasting, start cooking the couscous.

7. For Couscous: Heat olive oil in a skillet over medium heat, then add dried couscous. Stir and toast until golden brown, about 5-7 minutes. Meanwhile, heat 2.25 cups of water in a small pot until it boils.

8. Once boiling, add ½ teaspoon of kosher salt and toasted couscous. Turn the heat to medium, cover, and cook for 12-15 minutes, or until most of the water has evaporated. Drain as needed and set aside.

9. Once your vegetables have finished roasting, take them from the oven and carefully pull off the roasted garlic cloves. Press the garlic out of the skin and pour it over the remaining vegetables. It should have an extremely smooth texture.

10. Place everything in a large serving bowl and stir. Combine with cooked couscous and top with fresh parsley for garnish.

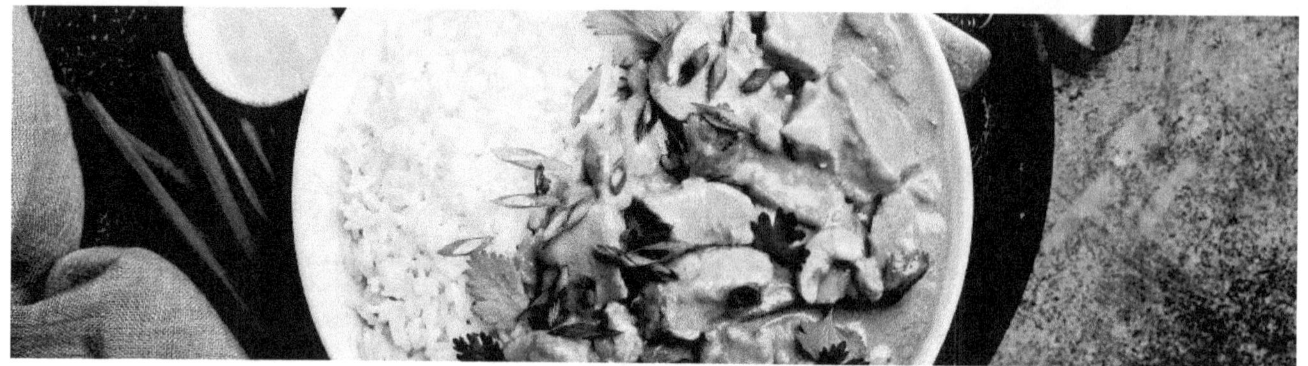

Chicken and Vegetable Curry with Rice

CALORIES: 355   **FAT: 11G**   **PROTEIN: 43G**   **CARB: 22G**

SERVINGS: 1   **PREP TIME: 15 MINS**   **COOK TIME: 35 MINS**

INGREDIENTS

2 tablespoons avocado or olive oil, split

Cut 1.25 pounds of chicken breast or thighs into 1-inch cubes.

Chop 1 cup yellow onion.

Mince 3 garlic cloves.

Finely chopped, peeled ginger (1 tablespoon)

3 carrots, peeled and cut into thin rings

One finely sliced red bell pepper

One medium zucchini, cut

1 ½ tablespoons yellow curry powder

Add 1 teaspoon paprika.

Add 1 ¼ teaspoon salt and more to taste.

1 13.5-ounce can coconut milk

1/2 cup vegetable or chicken broth.

Add black pepper to taste.

Use cilantro for serving.

Prepared basmati rice for serving.

DIRECTIONS

1. Heat 1 tablespoon of oil in a large skillet or Dutch oven over medium heat. Once the oil is hot, add the chicken chunks and sauté for 9-11 minutes, or until thoroughly cooked and browned. While the chicken is cooking, sprinkle it with a little salt and pepper. Once done, remove the chicken and set aside.
2. Add 1 tablespoon of oil to the same skillet. Sauté the onion, garlic, ginger, and carrots for about 5-7 minutes, or until fragrant and the carrots softened somewhat.
3. Cook for an additional 5 minutes with the red pepper and zucchini.
4. Stir in the curry powder, paprika, salt, coconut milk, and vegetable broth. Bring the mixture to a low boil. Once boiling, reduce the heat to a simmer for 10-15 minutes, or until the vegetables are cooked.
5. Return the chicken to the pan, stir, and cook for another 2-3 minutes, or until warmed through.
6. Season to taste, then serve over cooked rice and sprinkle with fresh cilantro.

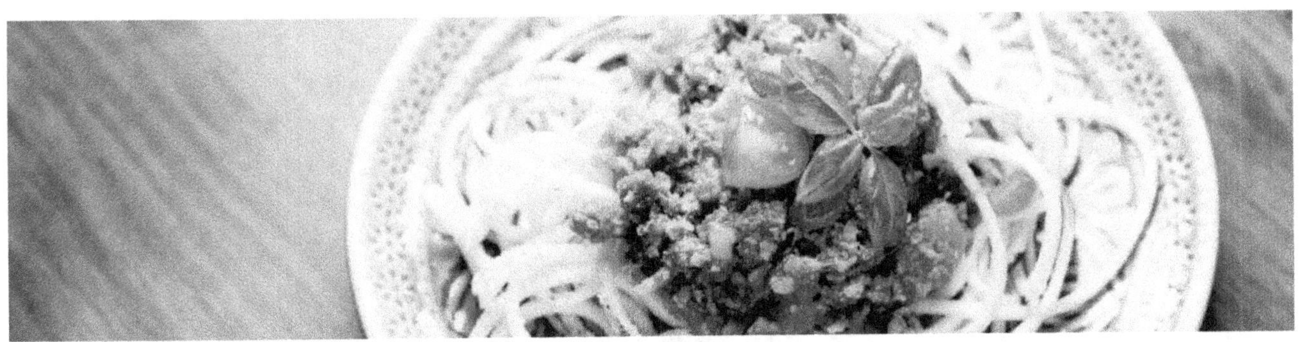

Zucchini noodles (Zoodles) with Marinara Sauce

CALORIES: 241　　**FAT: 18G**　　**PROTEIN: 7G**　　**CARB: 11G**

SERVINGS: 4　　**PREP TIME: 15 MINS**　　**COOK TIME: 20 MINS**

INGREDIENTS

4 tablespoons olive oil, divided.

6 cloves of garlic, minced

1 (28 ounces) can whole, peeled tomatoes

1 teaspoon of kosher salt.

1/2 teaspoon red pepper flakes.

¼ teaspoon dried oregano.

One huge sprig of basil

2 lb zucchini

Optional: 1/2 cup grated Parmesan cheese or minced fresh herbs.

DIRECTIONS

1. Heat 2 tablespoons of olive oil in a big pot or Dutch oven over medium-hServe the zucchini noodles covered with tomato sauce. Optional toppings include fresh herbs or a sprinkling of parmesan cheese.
2. igh heat. Once hot, add the garlic and sauté until it sizzles.
3. Before the garlic browns, combine the peeled tomatoes, salt, red pepper flakes, and oregano with 1 cup water. Bring to a low boil, then lower heat. Simmer for fifteen minutes. Stir occasionally and use a spoon to break up the larger bits of tomato
4. Add the sprig of basil to the sauce in the last 3 minutes of cooking, leaving the end sticking out so you can pull it out and discard it after the pasta is done.
5. Meanwhile, spiralize or ribbon the zucchini with a spiralizer or veggie peeler.
6. In a large skillet, heat a tablespoon of olive oil until hot. Add half of the zucchini noodles. Toss them to coat with oil and fry for 2 minutes. Remove and set aside. Heat the remaining tablespoon of oil and cook the remaining zucchini noodles.
7. In a large skillet, heat a tablespoon of olive oil until hot. Add half of the zucchini noodles. Toss them to coat with oil and fry for 2 minutes. Remove and set aside. Heat the remaining tablespoon of oil and cook the remaining zucchini noodles.
8. Serve the zucchini noodles covered with tomato sauce. Optional toppings include fresh herbs or a sprinkling of parmesan cheese.

86

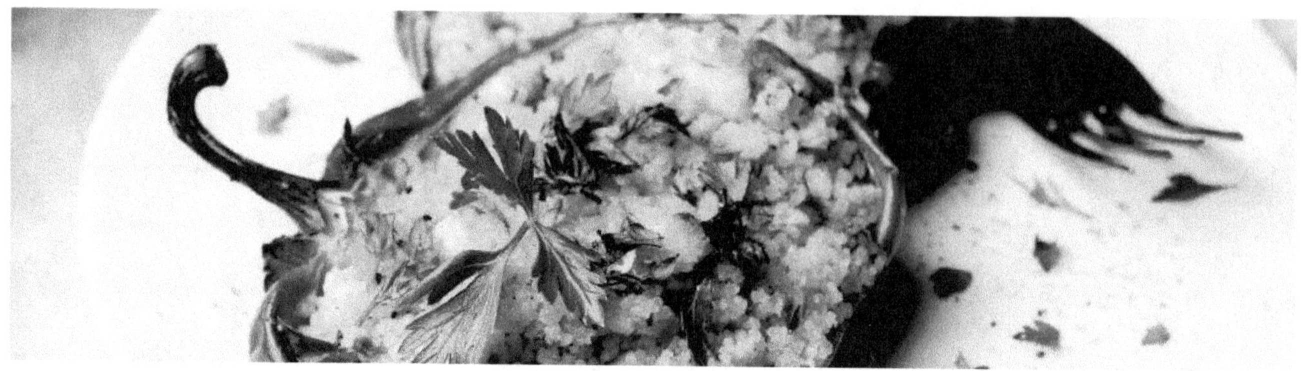

Taco-stuffed bell peppers with ground turkey

CALORIES: 175   **FAT: 34G**   **PROTEIN: 38G**   **CARB: 25G**

SERVINGS: 1   **PREP TIME: 15 MINS**   **COOK TIME: 25 MINS**

INGREDIENTS

4 bell peppers, split in half lengthwise and seeds removed.
2 tablespoons of olive oil.
½ teaspoon salt.
1/2 teaspoon freshly cracked black pepper.
½ teaspoon garlic powder.
1 tablespoon of olive oil.
1 bell pepper, diced
1 shallot, diced
1 lb. Shady Brook Farms 93% ground turkey
2 tablespoons ground cumin
2 teaspoons of smoked paprika.
1 teaspoon of chili powder.
½ teaspoon garlic powder.
1/2 teaspoon of salt.
1/2 teaspoon of freshly cracked pepper.
½ cup water
1 teaspoon of all-purpose flour.
Shredded sharp cheddar cheese, freshly grated.
Guacamole for serving.
Drizzle with taco sauce or salsa.
Fresh cilantro for serving.
Cotija cheese for serving.

DIRECTIONS

1. Preheat the oven to 400 degrees Fahrenheit. Brush the peppers (both inside and outside) with olive oil and season with salt, pepper, and garlic powder. Place the peppers on a baking sheet and roast for 15–20 minutes.
2. While the peppers roast, prepare the turkey taco meat. Place a large skillet over medium heat and add the olive oil. Combine the diced peppers, shallot, and garlic with a pinch of salt. Cook, stirring frequently, until softened, approximately 5 minutes.
3. Add the ground turkey and break it up with a wooden spoon. Season with cumin, paprika, chili powder, garlic powder, salt, and pepper. Stir well, breaking up the meat into small crumbs. Cook until the turkey is browned
4. Shake the water and flour in a shaker bottle for 30 seconds. Pour the mixture into the tacos, stirring well, and cook for an additional 5 to 6 minutes, or until saucy.
5. Remove the peppers from the oven. Fill the peppers with turkey taco mix.
6. At this point, you can cover with cheese, drizzle with taco sauce, or leave them alone! I like to put them back in the oven for about 15 minutes until everything comes together.
7. Top with guacamole, cilantro, and cotija cheese

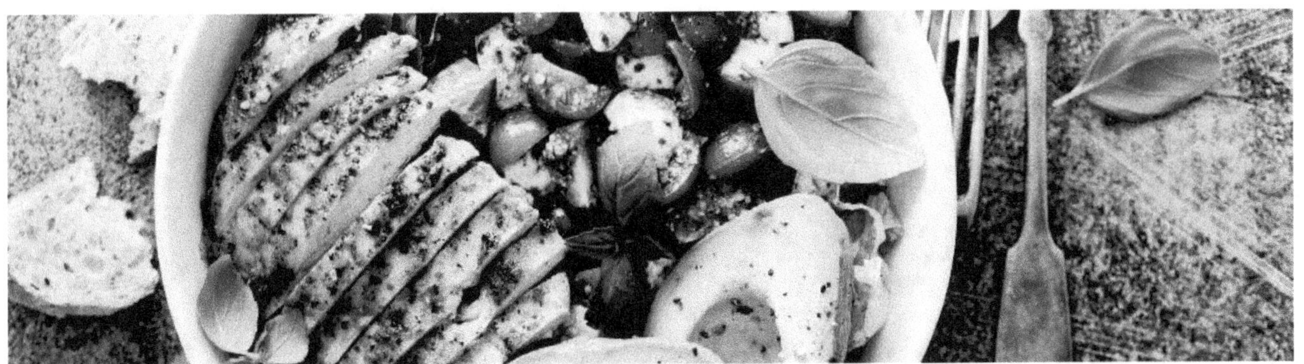

Pesto Chicken with Caprese Salad

CALORIES: 793   **FAT: 33G**   **PROTEIN: 62G**   **CARB: 22G**

SERVINGS: 1   **COOK TIME: 10 MINS**   **TOTAL TIME: 20 MINS**

INGREDIENTS

Pesto

1 cup firmly packed fresh basil leaves
from a 4-ounce container.
1/4 cup pine nuts
1/4 cup freshly grated Parmesan cheese
Add 1 to 3 cloves garlic to taste.
One teaspoon of lemon juice.
Add 1 teaspoon kosher salt, or more to
taste.
1/2 teaspoon freshly ground black
pepper, or to taste.
⅓ to ½ cup HemisFares Extra Virgin
Olive Oil.

Chicken

Add 2 teaspoons of HemisFares Extra
Virgin Olive Oil.
Dice 1 1/4 pounds boneless, skinless
chicken breast into bite-size
pieces.Add ½ teaspoon kosher salt or
to taste.
1/2 teaspoon freshly ground black
pepper, or to taste.
⅓ cup pesto.
Continue ■

DIRECTIONS

Make A Pesto:

1. Add the basil, pine nuts, parmesan,
garlic, lemon juice (which keeps the
pesto from oxidizing as soon), salt,
and pepper to the canister of a food
processor fitted with the S-blade, and
pulse briefly on high speed to break
down the ingredients.

2. With the motor running, drizzle in
the olive oil until the pesto is smooth
and emulsified. Set aside.

3..

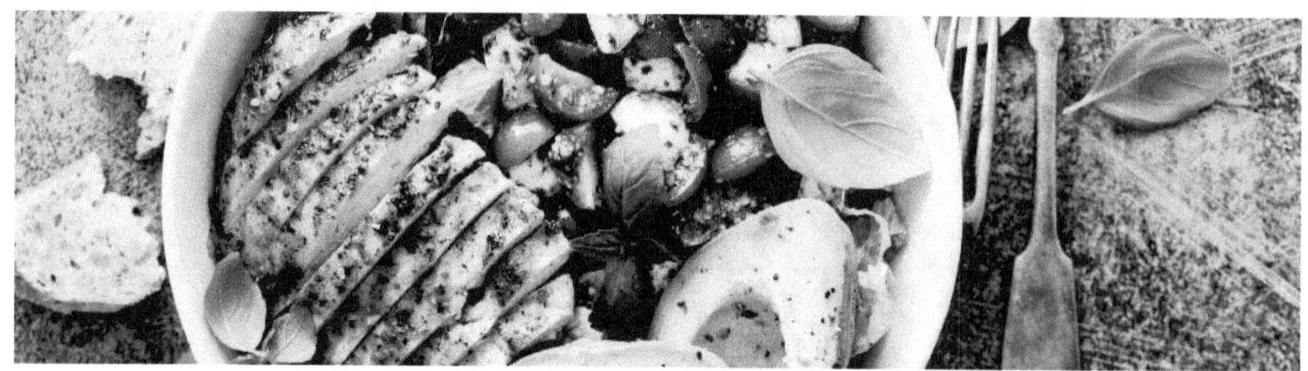

INGREDIENTS

CAPRESE SALAD.

1 ½ cup cherry or grape tomatoes, halved if desired.

Drain one 8-ounce container of fresh mozzarella 'pearls' or

little balls.

Tear roughly 10 fresh basil leaves in half.

Drizzle with 1 to 2 tablespoons of balsamic reduction or glaze

to taste.

DIRECTIONS

Make the chicken:

4. In a large skillet, combine the olive oil and chicken, season with salt and pepper, and cook over medium-high heat, stirring and flipping periodically to ensure uniform cooking.

5. When the chicken is about 90% cooked, toss in the pesto, reduce the heat to low, and let it simmer for about 2 to 3 minutes, or until done (internal temperature of 165F).

Assemble the caprese salad.

6. In a large bowl, combine the chicken, pesto/pan juices, mozzarella, and basil. Drizzle with balsamic and swirl to blend. Serve immediately. The dish is best served fresh

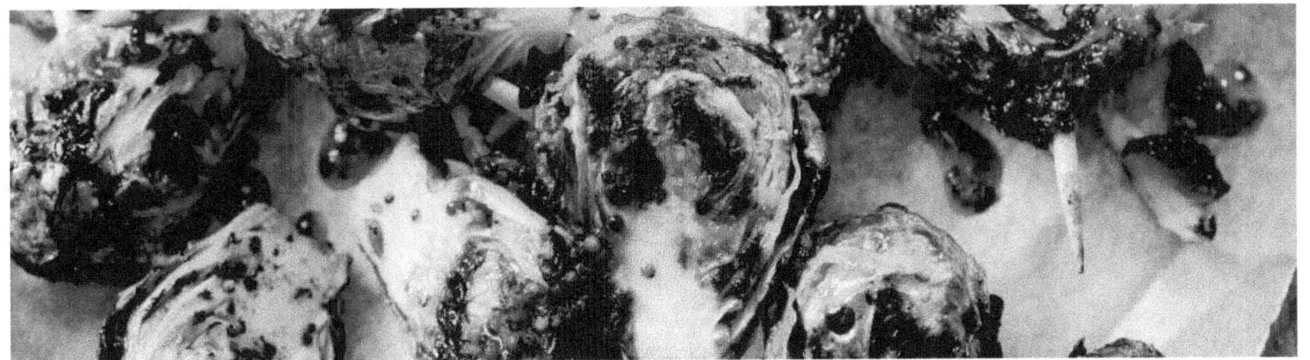

Honey Sriracha Glazed Roasted Brussels Sprouts

CALORIES: 114   **FAT: 4G**   **PROTEIN: 4G**   **CARB: 19G**

SERVINGS: 4   **PREP TIME: 5 MINS**   **COOK TIME: 25 MINS**

INGREDIENTS

One pound of fresh Brussels sprouts.

One tablespoon of extra virgin olive oil.

Add salt and pepper to taste.

Honey Sriracha Glaze

2 tablespoons of honey.

2 teaspoons sriracha.

Add 2 tablespoons of rice wine vinegar.

1 teaspoon Dijon mustard.

One teaspoon of soy sauce

DIRECTIONS

1. Preheat the oven to 400 °F. Trim any browned stems or leaves from the sprouts. Cut brussels sprouts lengthwise through the stem end. Line a baking sheet with foil or parchment paper and coat with cooking spray.
2. ROAST: Toss sliced Brussels sprouts in olive oil, season with salt and pepper to taste. Distribute them evenly on a baking sheet, cut side down. Roast for 20-30 minutes, until the inside is fork soft and the outside is crispy.
3. GLAZE: While the sprouts are in the oven, whisk together the glaze ingredients.
4. TOSS: Toss the roasted Brussels sprouts with the glaze and serve immediately.

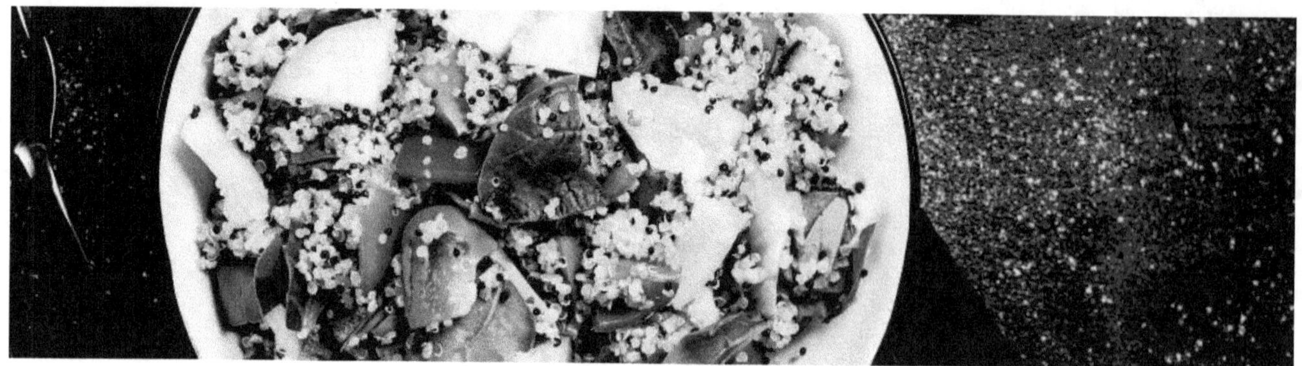

Vegetarian Quinoa Paella

CALORIES: 242   **FAT: 10G**   **PROTEIN: 6G**   **CARB: 30G**

SERVINGS: 6   **PREP TIME: 15 MINS**   **COOK TIME: 30 MINS**

INGREDIENTS

1 tablespoon of olive oil.

1 medium white onion, chopped.

2 - 3 garlic cloves minced

1 cup chopped baby bella mushrooms, approximately 6 - 8 mushrooms.

1 15-ounce can chickpeas, drained and rinsed.

1 14.5-ounce can chopped tomatoes (I used fire-roasted)

1 14.5-ounce can of artichoke hearts, in water

1 cup white quinoa.

1 teaspoon of smoked paprika.

1/2 teaspoon of saffron threads.

Salt and pepper to taste.

2 cups veggie broth.

1 cup of frozen green beans.

1 bell pepper, sliced

Optional: Juice from 1/2 lemon.

DIRECTIONS

1. Heat the oil in a large skillet over medium heat. Sauté onions and garlic until transparent, about 2 minutes. Cook for another 2 - 3 minutes, until the mushrooms begin to soften.

2. Once the mushrooms begin to brown, add the chickpeas, tomatoes, artichokes, quinoa, paprika, and saffron. Season with salt and pepper, then mix everything together. Add the broth and whisk again to combine. Bring the mixture to a boil, then cover and let it simmer for 20 - 25 minutes, or until the majority of the liquid is absorbed.

3. Remove the lid and add the green beans. Smooth the top of the paella with your spoon, then lay the sliced bell peppers on top. Cover again and cook for a further 10 minutes.

4. When ready to serve, pour lemon juice over the top and serve immediately!

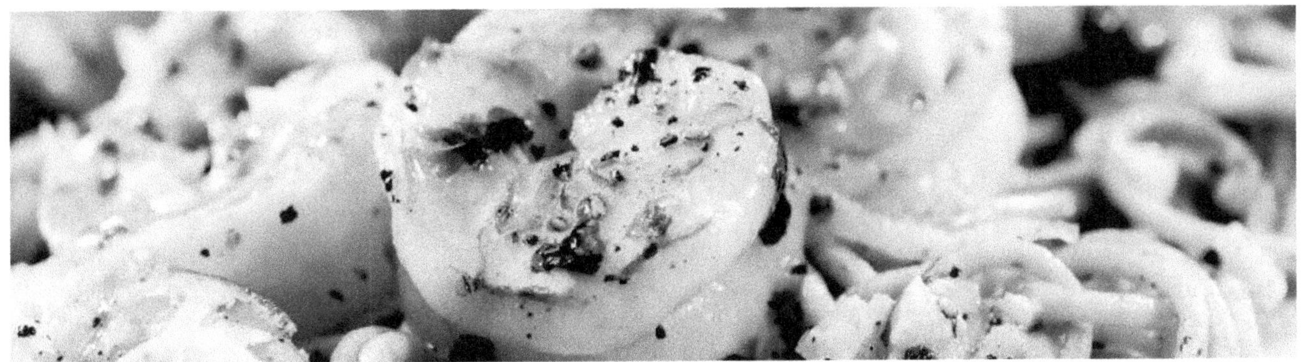

Lemon Garlic Shrimp with Asparagus

CALORIES: 302   **FAT: 19.5G**   **PROTEIN: 27G**   **CARB: 6.2G**

SERVINGS: 4   **PREP TIME: 5 MINS**   **COOK TIME: 15 MINS**

INGREDIENTS

For the shrimp:

1 lb medium-sized shrimp, peeled and deveined.
1 tablespoon olive oil.
1/4 cup melted butter.
3 tablespoons lemon juice.
1 teaspoon lemon zest.
Add 1 tablespoon minced garlic.
Add 1/2 teaspoon paprika.
1/4 teaspoon onion powder.
1/4 tsp red pepper flakes, optional if you prefer less heat.
Add salt and pepper to taste.
Add fresh parsley as garnish after cooking.

For the Asparagus:

1 pound thin to medium asparagus with clipped ends
1 tablespoon olive oil.
Mince 2 cloves of garlic.
1 teaspoon lemon zest.
Add salt and pepper to taste.

DIRECTIONS

1. Preheat the oven to 400 degrees Fahrenheit.
2. In a large bowl, combine the olive oil, melted butter, lemon juice, zest, garlic, and spices.
3. Toss in the shrimp and mix until evenly coated. Set aside and marinade the shrimp while the asparagus cooks.
4. Arrange asparagus on one side of a big sheet pan greased with nonstick spray. Drizzle with olive oil and season with garlic and lemon zest.
5. Toss until evenly coated, then season with salt and pepper. Place in the oven and cook for 5 minutes.
6. Once the asparagus has finished cooking, remove it from the oven and arrange the marinated shrimp on the other side of the pan in a single layer. Place everything back in the oven and cook for another 8 to 10 minutes, or until the shrimp are opaque and pink.
7. Remove from the oven, squeeze in more lemon juice, and sprinkle with fresh parsley.
8. Enjoy!

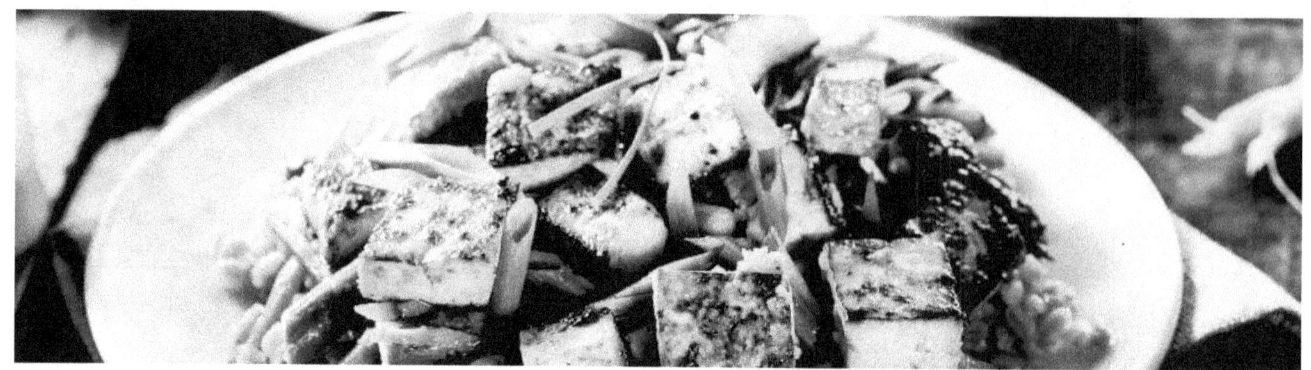

Cauliflower Fried Rice With Tofu

CALORIES: 259　　　**FAT: 12G**　　　**PROTEIN: 17G**　　　**CARB: 25G**

SERVINGS: 1　　　**PREP TIME: 10 MINS**　　　**TOTAL TIME: 10 MINS**

INGREDIENTS

Add 2 tablespoons of toasted sesame oil.

One block of exceptionally firm tofu

Use 12 oz frozen or fresh cauliflower rice.

1 lb frozen vegetable mix including carrots, peas, corn, and green peas.

2 eggs, lightly beaten

1/2 medium onion, chopped.

Optional: 1 teaspoon garlic and chili paste.

Divide three tablespoons of low-sodium soy sauce, tamari, or coconut aminos.

Finely dice or smash two peeled garlic cloves.

1 inch ginger, grated or minced

Add salt and pepper to taste.

DIRECTIONS

1. Press the tofu. Take the tofu out of the package, drain it, cover it in a clean cotton cloth or paper towels, and set it on a dish with something heavy on top. If you own a tofu press, use it instead. Keep it squeezed for at least 15 minutes to remove most of the moisture.

2. Place the dried tofu on a chopping board and cut it into cubes or rectangles. I like to cut the mu tofu into 2-inch rectangles, but it's up to you.

3. In a medium bowl, whisk together 2 tablespoons soy sauce (tamari or coconut aminos), 1 tablespoon toasted sesame oil, and 1 teaspoon garlic-chili paste (if using). Use a silicone spatula to coat the tofu blocks, being careful not to break them. If you have time or are planning ahead of time, let the tofu marinate in the fridge for 15 minutes to a couple of hours. If you are short on time, you can skip this step and cook the tofu immediately.

4. ....

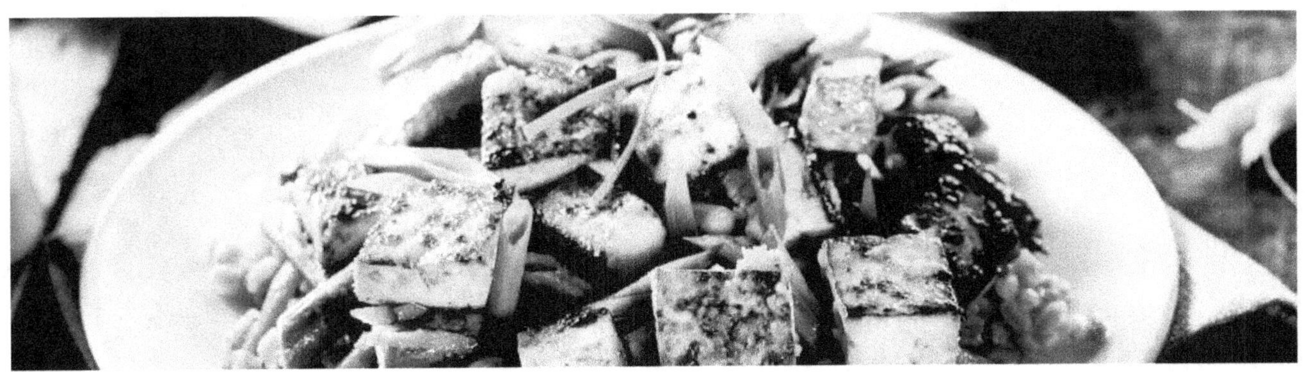

DIRECTIONS

1. Bake or air fried tofu. If baking in the oven, place the tofu on a large baking sheet lined with parchment paper or sprayed with nonstick spray and bake at 425 degrees Fahrenheit for about 30 minutes, flipping once after 15 minutes. If you have an air fryer, set it to 375 degrees Fahrenheit. Spray the bottom of the basket with nonstick spray and arrange the tofu blocks in a single layer. Cook for 10-15 minutes, shaking the pan occasionally to ensure equal frying. It should be crispy on the outside.

2. Prepare the fried cauliflower rice while the tofu bakes or air fries. Heat the remaining 1 tablespoon sesame oil in a large skillet, then add the onion and cook for a minute or two until softened. Add the garlic and ginger and stir cook for another minute, or until fragrant.

3. Cook the frozen vegetable mix and cauliflower rice on medium heat, turning frequently, until the veggies are tender, about 5 minutes. If using fresh cauliflower rice, add it a few minutes after the frozen veggie mixture and incorporate. Fresh cauliflower rice will require less time to prepare.

4. Make a well in the center of the vegetable mixture, heat to medium-high, add the gently beaten eggs, and scramble with a spatula until the eggs are no longer liquid. Stir into the cauliflower-vegetable mixture. Add 1 tablespoon soy sauce, mix, and taste. Season with salt and pepper, then add additional soy sauce (tamari or coconut aminos) as necessary.

5. Spoon the stir fry into dishes and top with crispy tofu.

6. Optional toppings include chopped cilantro or spring onions, toasted sesame seeds, and a sprinkle of Sriracha.

APPETIZERS

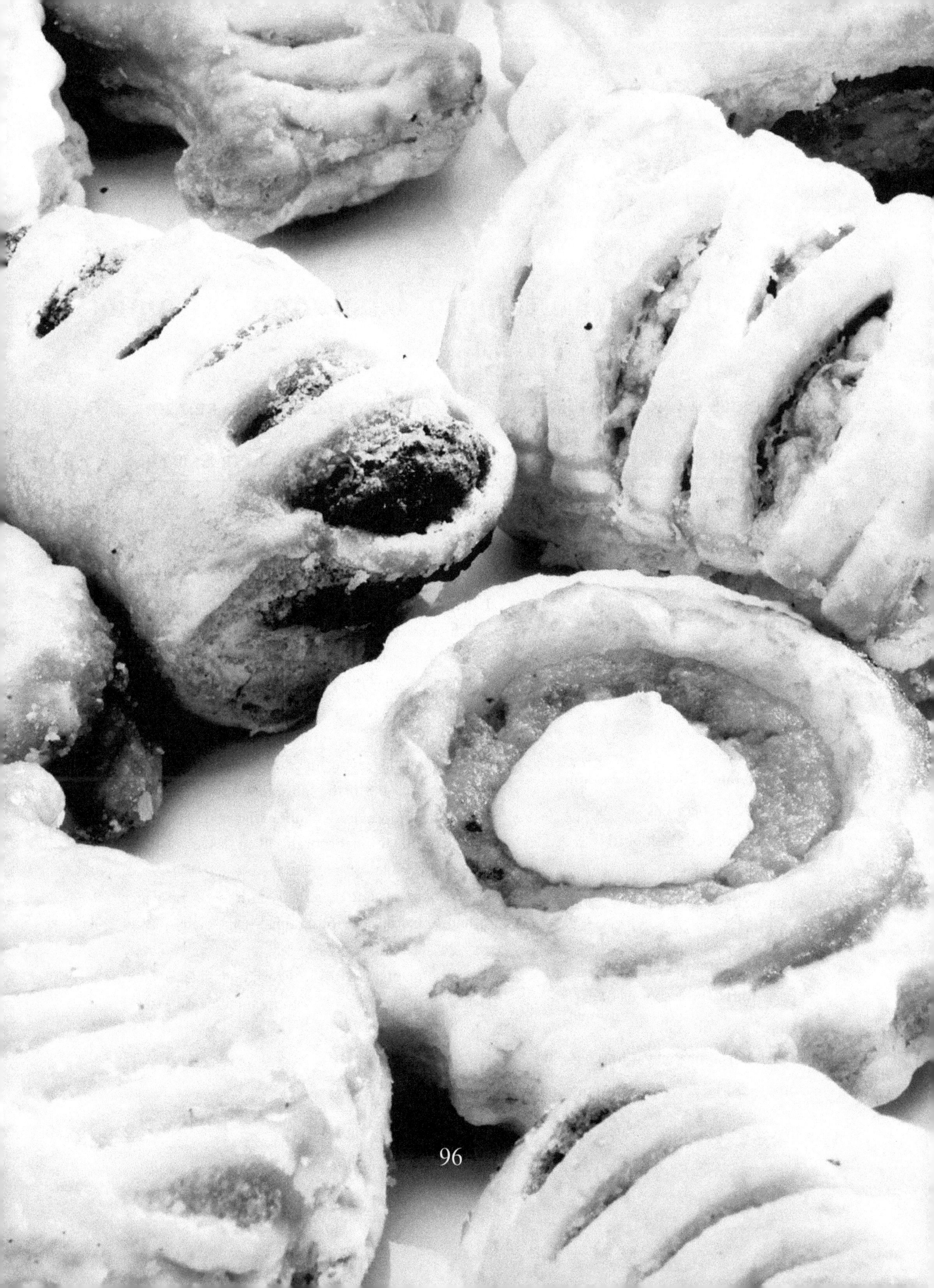

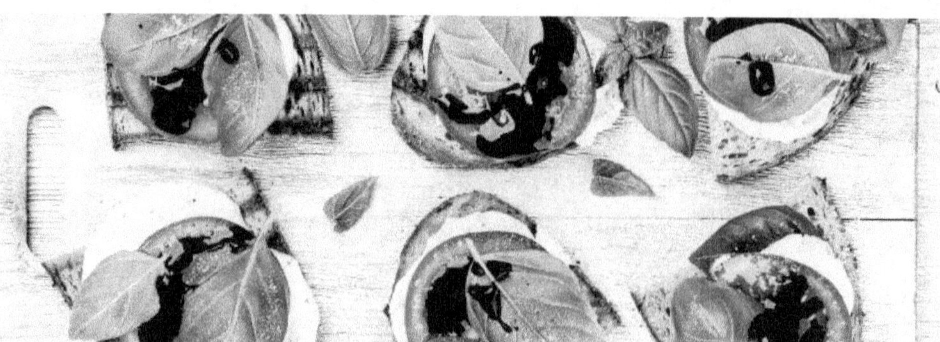

Bruschetta with tomato, basil, and balsamic glaze.

CALORIES: 64　　**FAT: 1.2G**　　**PROTEIN: 1.6G**　　**CARB:7.7G**

SERVINGS: 24　　**PREP TIME: 31 MINS**　　**COOK TIME: 10 MINS**

INGREDIENTS

2 pounds of ripe tomatoes (approximately 5 to 6 medium tomatoes, although any type would do)

1/2 teaspoon fine sea salt, plus more to taste.

1/2 cup finely sliced white onion (approx. ½ medium)

½ cup chopped fresh basil (about. ¾ ounce)

2 garlic cloves, crushed or minced.

One baguette (French bread).

Four to five tablespoons of extra virgin olive oil, split

Thick balsamic vinegar and optional Maldon flaky sea salt

DIRECTIONS

1. Preheat your oven (or gas grill*) to 450 degrees Fahrenheit. For easier cleanup, line a big, rimmed baking sheet with parchment paper. If your baking sheet is smaller than mine, you may need to make the toast in two separate batches.

2. Dice the tomatoes and transfer to a medium mixing bowl, leaving the seeds and liquid on the cutting board. Stir the salt into the tomatoes, then add the onion, basil, and garlic when they are ready. Stir to incorporate, then leave away to marinate while you prepare the bread.

3. Cut your baguette diagonally into pieces no wider than ½-inch (see photographs). I normally put 20 to 24 slices on my large baking sheet; you may have some bread leftover. Brush both sides of each slice with olive oil (approximately 2 to 3 teaspoons).

4. ......

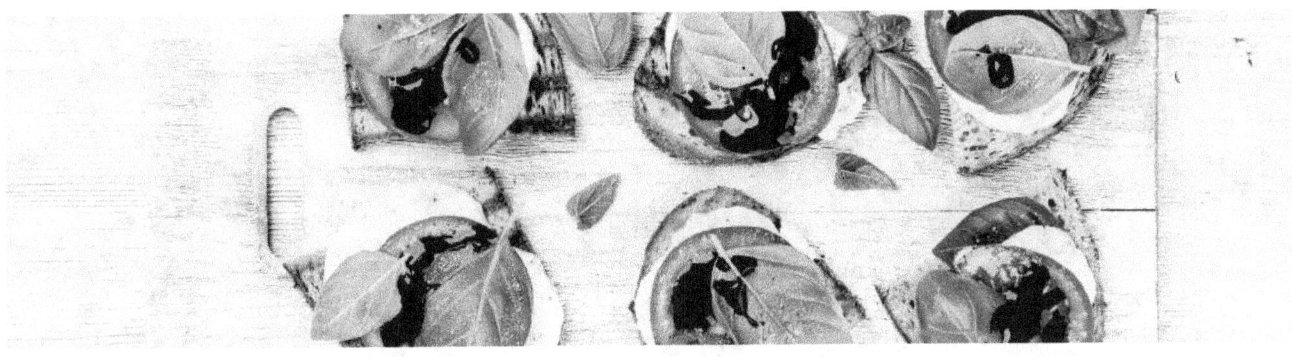

DIRECTIONS

4. Place the slices in a single layer on the prepared baking sheet and bake for 6 to 9 minutes on the middle rack, or until crisp and golden. If preferred, transfer the toasts to one or more serving platters and leave aside

5. When you're ready to serve, carefully drain off any excess tomato juice that has accumulated in the bowl, using your hand as a stopper. Add the remaining 2 tbsp olive oil. Mix well and season with salt to taste (I generally put ¼ to ½ teaspoon). If you don't think your bruschetta is garlicky enough (I prefer my mildly but not overly garlicky), add another crushed clove of garlic.

6. Top each bread with the tomato mixture, tipping your spoon against the bowl to expel any excess juice. Drizzle a couple of tablespoons of thick balsamic vinegar over the top, then sprinkle with flaky salt if you have any. Bruschetta is best served quickly.

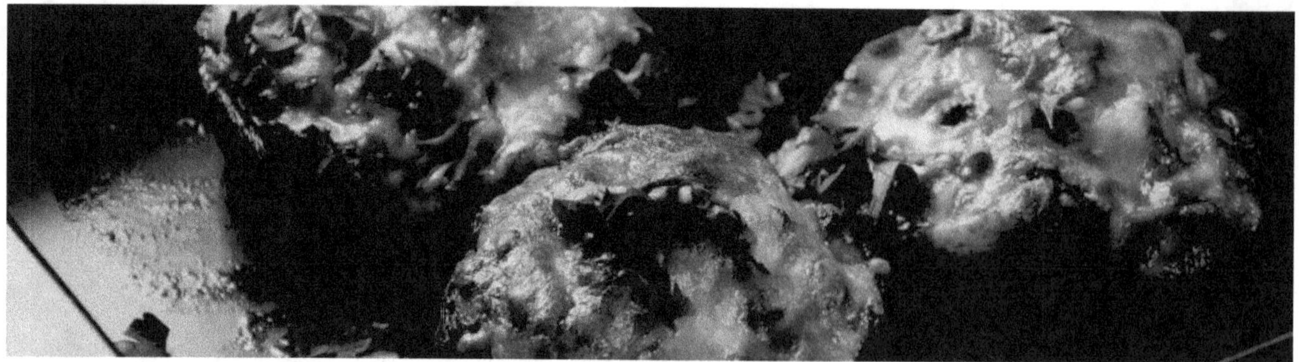

Stuffed Mushrooms With Cream Cheese And Garlic

CALORIES: 176   **FAT: 16G**   **PROTEIN: 5G**   **CARB: 3G**

SERVINGS: 6   **PREP TIME: 15 MINS**   **COOK TIME: 35 MINS**

INGREDIENTS

Cooking Spray

12 entire fresh mushrooms with tough ends cut.

1 tablespoon of vegetable oil.

1 tablespoon of minced garlic.

1 (8-ounce) box of softened cream cheese

¼ cup grated Parmesan

1/4 teaspoon ground black pepper

¼ teaspoon onion powder.

¼ teaspoon cayenne pepper

DIRECTIONS

1. Preheat the oven to 350 degrees Fahrenheit/175 degrees Celsius. Spray a baking sheet with cooking spray.
2. Clean the mushrooms with a moist paper towel. Carefully remove the stems from the mushrooms. Finely cut the stems and set the caps aside.
3. Heat the oil in a large skillet over medium heat. Fry chopped mushroom stems and garlic in heated oil until any moisture has evaporated, 3 to 5 minutes, being careful not to burn the garlic. Spread the mushroom mixture into a bowl and let it cool fully, about 10 minutes.
4. Mix the cream cheese, Parmesan cheese, black pepper, onion powder, and cayenne pepper into the cooled mushroom mixture until well combined. Using a small spoon, generously fill each mushroom cap with stuffing. Arrange the stuffed mushrooms on the prepared cookie sheet.
5. Bake in a preheated oven for about 20 minutes, or until piping hot and liquid forms beneath each cap.

99

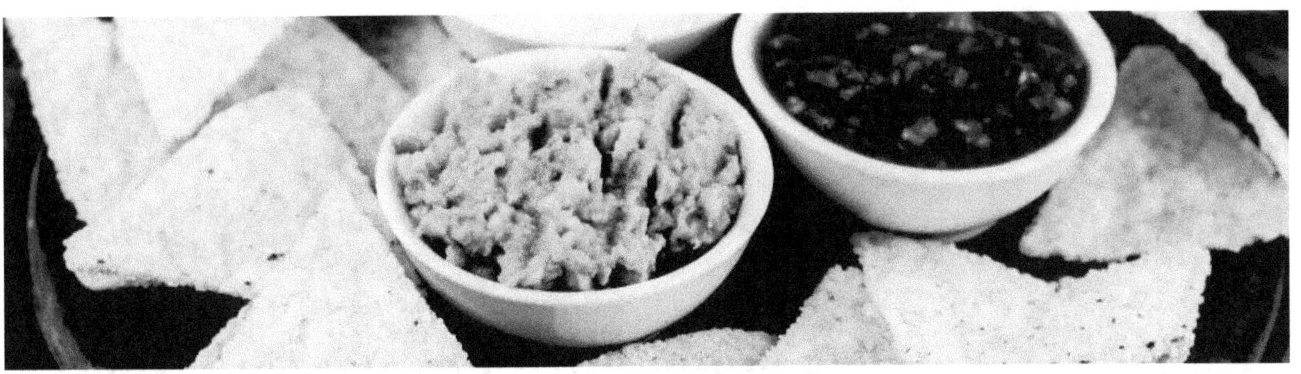

Guacamole with Tortilla Chips

CALORIES: 57   **FAT: 2.6G**   **PROTEIN: 1.2G**   **CARB: 8.3G**

SERVINGS: 16   **PREP TIME: 10 MINS**   **TOTAL TIME: 10 MINS**

INGREDIENTS

Chips:

Eight (6-inch) corn tortillas.

Cooking spray

½ teaspoon salt.

1/2 teaspoon chipotle chile powder

Guacamole:

3 tomatillos

⅓ cup diced onion

⅓ cup chopped plum tomatoes

3 tablespoons of chopped fresh cilantro.

1 tablespoon of fresh lime juice.

¾ teaspoon salt.

2 ripe, peeled avocados, seeds and coarsely mashed.

Seed and finely slice two jalapeño peppers.

One garlic clove, minced

DIRECTIONS

1. Preheat the oven to 375°.
2. To make chips, cut each tortilla into eight wedges and put them in a single layer on two baking pans covered with cooking spray. Sprinkle wedges with 1/2 teaspoon salt and chile powder, then lightly coat with cooking spray. Bake at 375° for 12 minutes, or until the wedges are crisp and lightly browned. Cool for 10 minutes.
3. To make guacamole, remove the papery husk from tomatillos; wash, core, and coarsely slice. Combine the tomatillos, onion, and remaining ingredients; mix well. Serve the guacamole with chips.

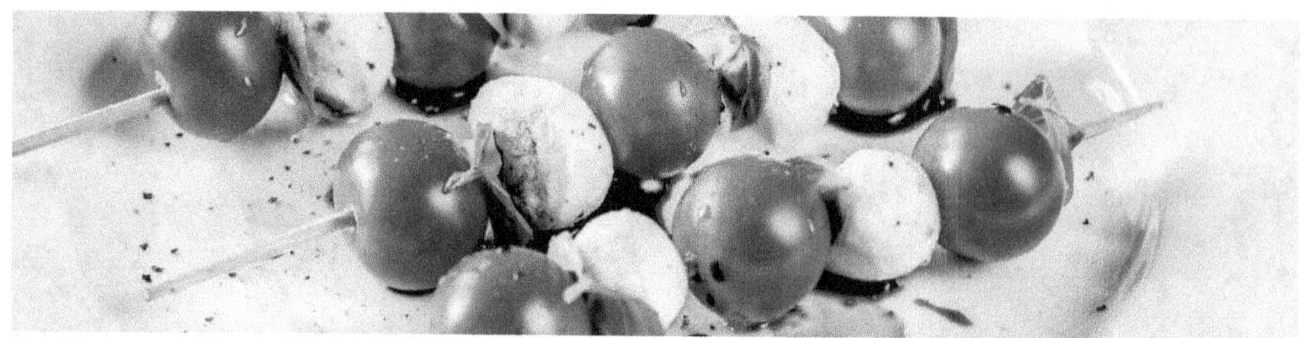

Caprese Skewers made with cherry tomatoes, mozzarella, and basil

CALORIES: 104   **FAT: 7G**   **PROTEIN: 7G**   **CARB: 2G**

SERVINGS: 1   **PREP TIME: 15 MINS**   **TOTAL TIME: 15 MINS**

INGREDIENTS

20 grape tomatoes.

10 ounces mozzarella cheese, cubed

2 tablespoons of extra virgin olive oil.

2 teaspoons of fresh basil leaves, chopped

1 pinch of salt.

1 pinch of ground black pepper.

Twenty toothpicks.

DIRECTIONS

1. Gather all the ingredients

2. Toss tomatoes, mozzarella cheese, olive oil, basil, salt, and pepper in a mixing bowl until well combined.

3. Skewer one tomato and one piece of mozzarella cheese onto each toothpick.

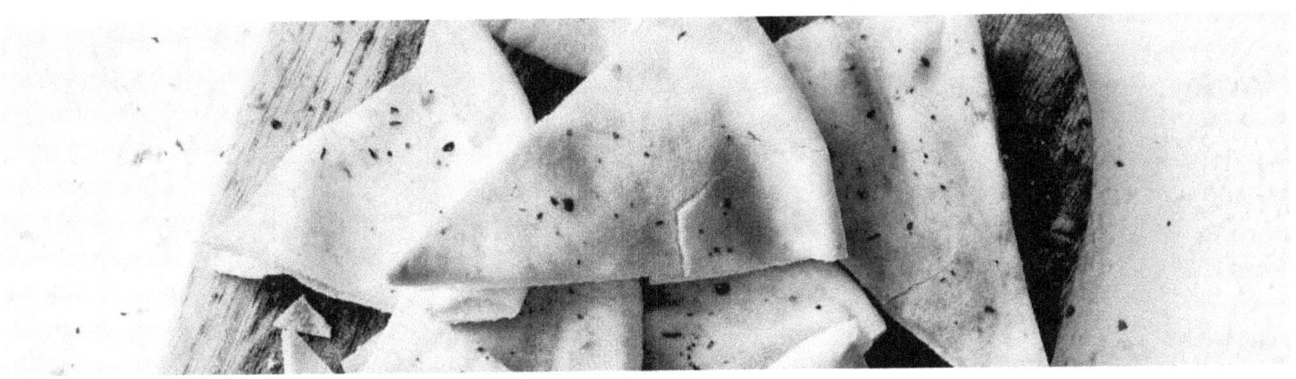

Pita Chips

CALORIES: 130   **FAT: 4G**   **PROTEIN: 3G**   **CARB: 20G**

SERVINGS: 8   **PREP TIME: 15 MINS**   **COOK TIME: 15 MINS**

INGREDIENTS

1 packet of pita pockets

2 tablespoons of olive oil.

1 tablespoon of garlic powder.

1 teaspoon of kosher salt.

1 teaspoon of garlic salt.

DIRECTIONS

1. Preheat the oven to 350 degrees Fahrenheit/175 degrees Celsius.
2. Brush one side of each pita pocket with olive oil, then season with garlic powder, salt, and garlic salt. Cut each pocket into four even triangles and place them, oiled side up, on a baking sheet.
3. Bake in a preheated oven for 15 to 20 minutes, or until the pita chips are light brown.

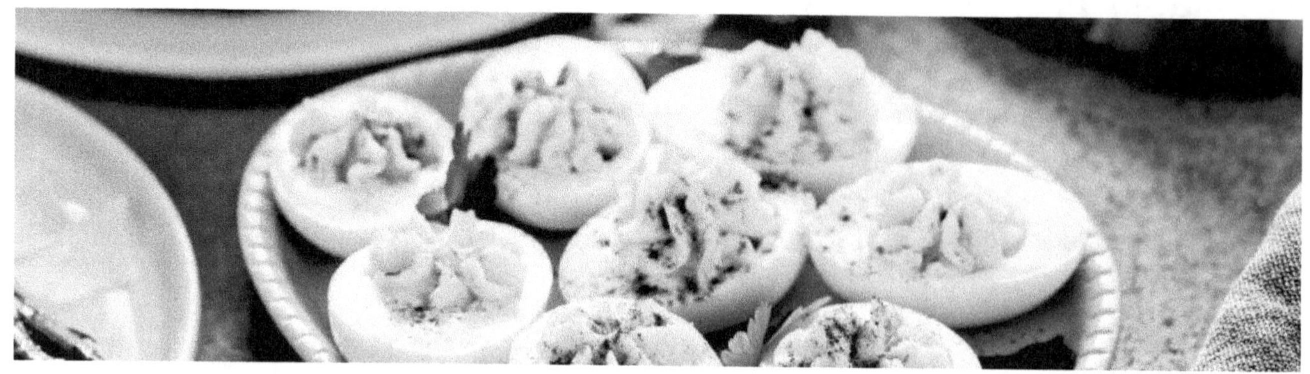

Deviled eggs with smoked paprika

CALORIES: 119   **FAT: 10.5G**   **PROTEIN: 13G**   **CARB: 1.1G**

SERVINGS: 12   **PREP TIME: 20 MINS**   **COOK TIME: 10 MINS**

INGREDIENTS

One dozen eggs.

Approximately 1/3 cup.

Hellmann's Mayonnaise (I use Canola Oil, which has less fat.)

About 1 tablespoon. Dry mustard

Fresh ground black pepper, to taste.

Good quality smoked paprika for garnish.

DIRECTIONS

1. Put entire eggs in a saucepan and just cover with cold water.
2. Cover them and turn your burner to high heat.
3. After the eggs have cooked, turn off the heat and let them stand for 10 minutes, covered.
4. Run cold water over the eggs without draining the hot water until the water in the pan is quite cold.
5. Allow the eggs to sit in the cool water for approximately 20 minutes. It is better to peel them immediately after cooling. If you aren't using them right away, put them in a closed container in the refrigerator for up to two days.
6. ......

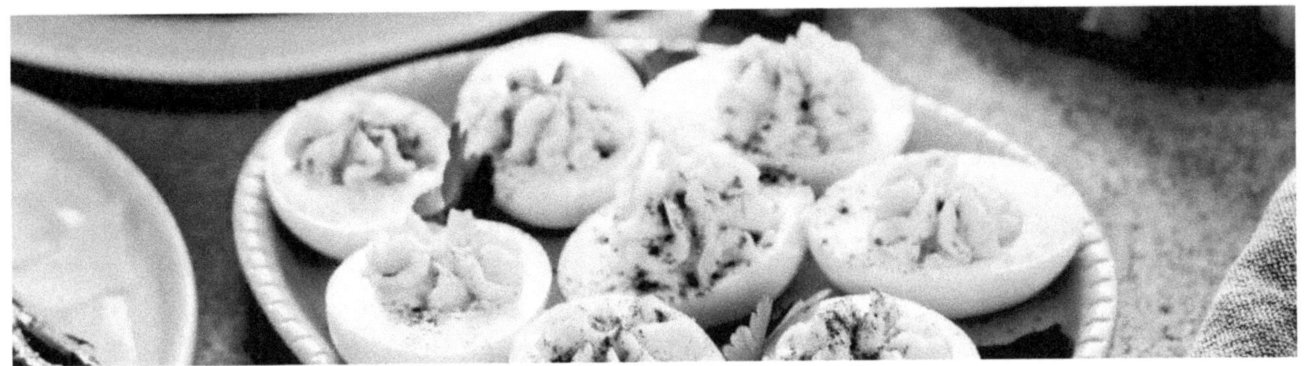

DIRECTIONS

6. Allow the eggs to sit in the cool water for approximately 20 minutes. It is better to peel them immediately after cooling. If you aren't using them right away, put them in a closed container in the refrigerator for up to two days.

7. Cut the eggs in half, then gently 'bend' each half with your thumbs on the spherical part of the egg. The yolks will usually slip right out. Put the yolks in a basin.

8. Once all of the yolks have been taken, mash them with a fork. I like to leave a few bits, but if you prefer a smooth filling, just keep mashing.

9. Combine the mayonnaise, dry mustard, and pepper, mixing fully but gently.

10. Cut a small corner from a plastic food storage bag for filling.

11. Fill the bag with the yolk mixture and pipe it into the holes in the egg white.

12. Once all of the eggs have been stuffed, sprinkle with smoked paprika.

13. Cover loosely with plastic wrap and chill until needed.

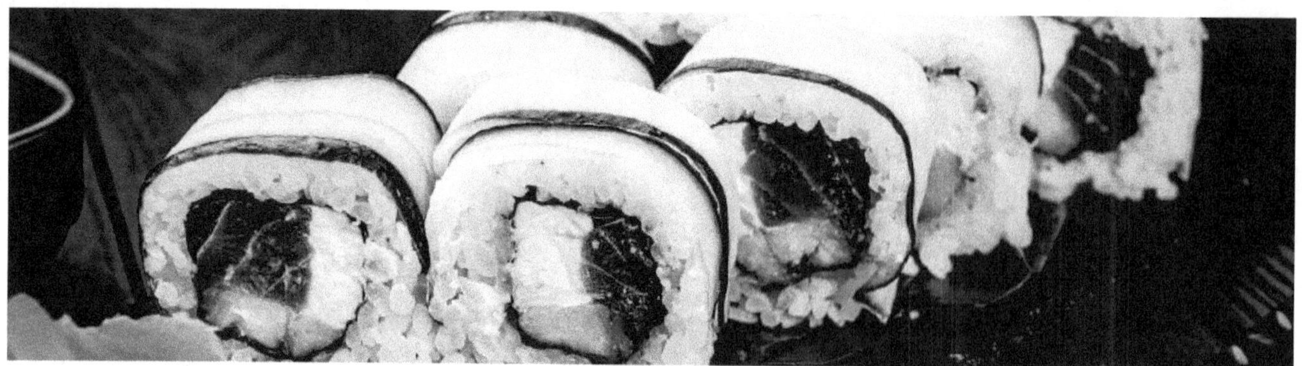

Cucumber Rolls with Herbal Cream Cheese

CALORIES: 78

SERVINGS: 1   **PREP TIME: 10 MINS**   **TOTAL TIME: 10 MINS**

INGREDIENTS

1 medium cucumber, thinly cut
horizontally (a vegetable peeler works
great here)

Cut 1 bell pepper, ½ orange, ½ yellow, or
any other color into small, thin strips.

Sliced avocado

For the Herbal Cream Cheese Spread:

4 ounces cream cheese at room
temperature.

1/2 teaspoon apple cider vinegar.

Pinch of salt.

A pinch of cayenne pepper.

1 sprig fresh dill, freshly chopped

1 sprig fresh flat-leafed parsley, coarsely
chopped

Optional: swap or add more of your
favorite herbs, such as fresh basil,
marjoram, and tarragon.

DIRECTIONS

1. Spread thinly sliced cucumber slices across a
   flat surface. Blot them carefully with dry
   paper towels to absorb any excess moisture.
   Set aside.

2. To make the herb cream cheese spread,
   whisk the room temperature cream cheese,
   apple cider vinegar, salt, and cayenne
   pepper until well combined. Add the finely
   chopped fresh herbs and stir to incorporate.

3. Spread a thin layer of herb cream cheese on
   each cucumber strip. Place your filling
   selections on one end of the cucumber (bell
   pepper strips, sliced avocado, or any other
   option you want!). Optional: Garnish with a
   little sprig of any fresh herb for display.

4. Roll it up and serve chilled.

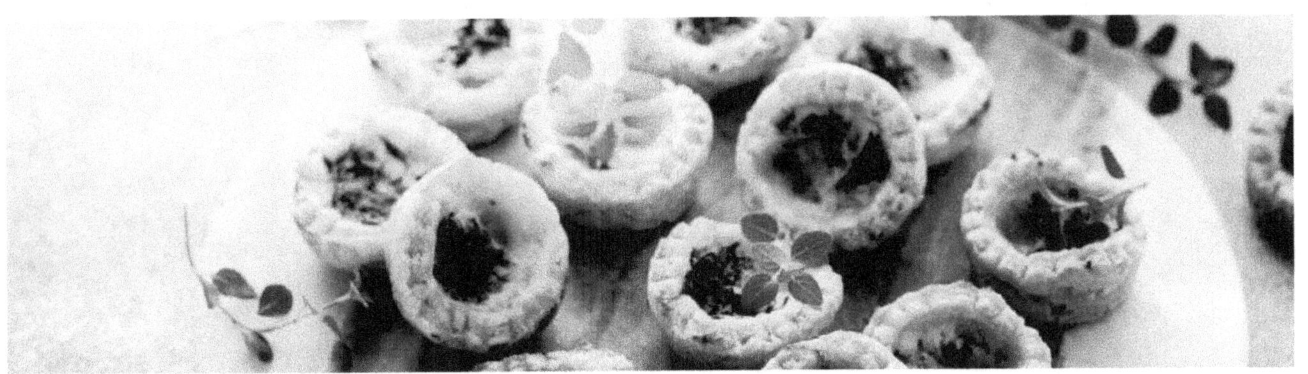

Mini quiche with spinach and feta

CALORIES: 385   **FAT: 27G**   **PROTEIN: 10G**   **CARB: 26G**

SERVINGS: 18   **PREP TIME: 20 MINS**   **COOK TIME: 18 MINS**

INGREDIENTS

Thawed 4 sheets of puff pastry.

100g baby spinach leaves.

90g of delicious cheese (1 cup)

½ cup parmesan cheese, 50 grams

100g crumbled feta

8 eggs

½ cup of milk (130 grams)

One tablespoon onion flakes.

Half teaspoon salt

1/4 teaspoon pepper.

DIRECTIONS

1. Preheat the oven to 200 degrees Celsius (fan forced).
2. Remove the pastry from the freezer and let it thaw slightly.
3. Grate the delicious and parmesan cheeses and reserve till required.
4. In a large jug, combine the milk, eggs, onion flakes, and salt and pepper.
5. Lightly grease two muffin tins, then cut circles of pastry with a 12 cm round cookie cutter and carefully mold them into the muffin tins - you'll create about 18 quiches.
6. ....

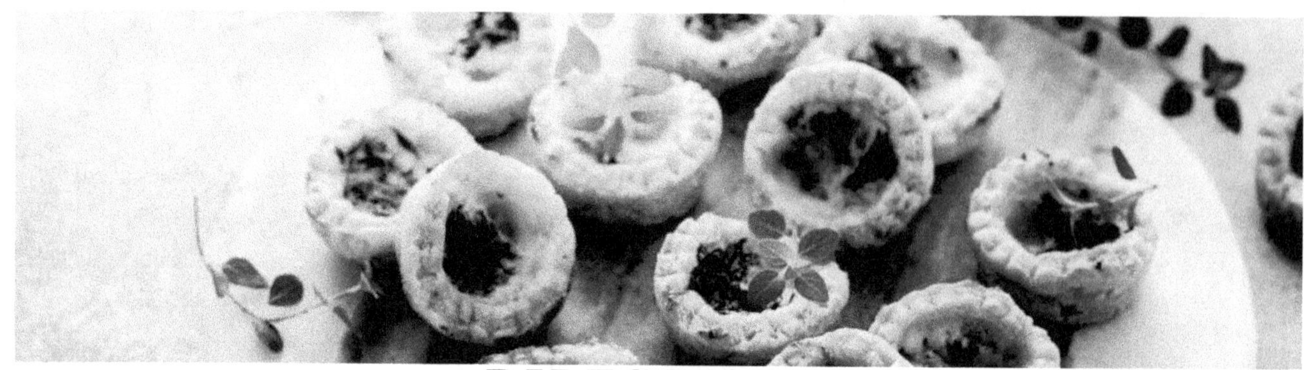

DIRECTIONS

7. Divide the young spinach leaves, feta, delicious, and parmesan cheese evenly between the pastry casings, then gently pour in the egg and milk mixture.

8. Place the two oven pans in the preheated oven and bake for 18 minutes, or until the filling is brown.

Allow the tiny quiches in the trays for 5 minutes to cool slightly before transferring to a wire rack to cool entirely.

THERMOMIX INSTRUCTIONS:

9. Preheat the oven to 200 degrees Celsius (fan forced).

10. Remove the pastry from the freezer and let it thaw slightly.

11. Place the parmesan and delicious cheese (cut into 3cm cubes) in your Thermomix bowl and grate for 7 seconds on speed 8.

12. Combine the milk, eggs, onion flakes, salt, and pepper by mixing for 10 seconds on speed 4.

13. crape down the sides of the basin and mix in the crumbled feta cheese.

14. Lightly grease two muffin tins, then cut circles of pastry with a 12 cm round cookie cutter and carefully mold them into the muffin tins - you'll create about 18 quiches.

15. Divide the young spinach leaves evenly between the pastry cases, then carefully pour in the mixture.

16. Place the two oven pans in the preheated oven and bake for 18 minutes, or until the filling is brown.

17. Leave the tiny quiches in the trays for 5 minutes to cool slightly before transferring to a wire rack to cool completely.

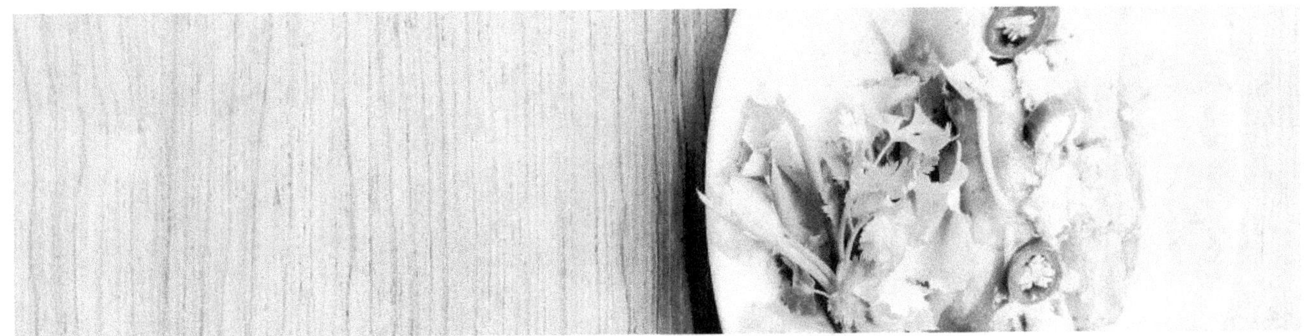

Vegetable Spring Rolls With Peanut Dipping Sauce

CALORIES: 177   **FAT: 8G**   **PROTEIN: 3.5G**   **CARB: 13.2G**

SERVINGS: 8   **PREP TIME: 40 MINS**   **COOK TIME: 5 MINS**

INGREDIENTS

Spring Rolls

2 oz rice vermicelli or brown rice noodles
1 teaspoon of toasted sesame oil.
¼ teaspoon fine sea salt
1 cup torn butter lettuce with ribs removed.
1 cup finely sliced red cabbage.
Two medium carrots, peeled and cut into matchsticks or strips with a julienne peeler.
2 Persian (mini) cucumbers or 1 small cucumber, thinly sliced or cut into strips using a julienne peeler.
Remove the ribs and seeds from two medium jalapeños and thinly slice them.
1/4 cup finely sliced green onions.
¼ cup finely chopped fresh cilantro
¼ cup finely chopped fresh mint
Eight sheets of rice paper (spring roll wrappers)

peanut sauce

⅓ cup creamy peanut butter.
2 teaspoons of rice vinegar.
2 tablespoons of reduced-sodium tamari or soy sauce.
Two teaspoons of honey or maple syrup
1 tablespoon of toasted sesame oil.
2 garlic cloves, crushed or minced.
2 to 3 tablespoons of water, as needed.

DIRECTIONS

1. To make the spring rolls, bring a pot of water to a boil and cook the noodles until al dente, following package recommendations. Drain, rinse with cool water, and then return to the saucepan. Turn off the heat and stir the noodles with the sesame oil and salt.
2. Fill a shallow pan (such as a pie pan or 9-inch circular cake pan) with an inch of water. Fold a lint-free tea towel in half and set it beside the plate. Make sure your prepared fillings are within reach. In a small bowl, combine the green onions, cilantro, and mint. Stir.
3. Put one rice paper in the water and let it sit for about 20 seconds, give or take. You'll learn to go by feel here—wait until the sheet is pliable but not overly floppy. Carefully place it flat on the towel.
4. Cover the lower third of the rice paper with butter lettuce, rice noodles, cabbage, carrot, cucumber, and jalapeño, leaving about 1 inch of space around the edges. Sprinkle generously with the herb mixture.
5. Fold the lower border up over the fillings and roll up just until the filling is completely encased. Fold the short sides over to form a burrito-style wrap. Finally, roll it up. Repeat with the remaining ingredients.
6. In a small mixing bowl, combine the peanut butter, rice vinegar, tamari, honey, sesame oil, and garlic. Whisk in 2 to 3 tablespoons of water as needed to create a creamy but dippable sauce.
7. Serve the spring rolls with peanut sauce on the side. You can serve them whole or cut in half diagonally with a sharp chef's knife.

108

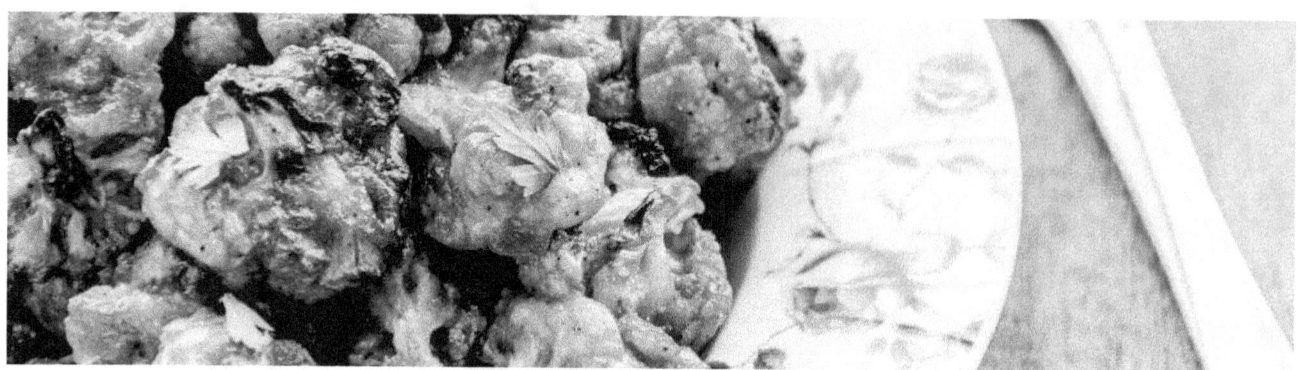

Baked Buffalo Cauliflower Bites

CALORIES: 127	**FAT: 3G**	**PROTEIN: 4G**	**CARB: 21G**
SERVINGS: 4	**PREP TIME: 10 MINS**	**COOK TIME: 40 MINS**	

INGREDIENTS

1 large head of cauliflower, chopped into florets

1/2 cup all-purpose flour.

Half cup water

Add 2 tablespoons of garlic powder.

Add 1 teaspoon paprika.

Half teaspoon salt

1/4 teaspoon of black pepper

Cooking Spray

1/2 cup hot sauce.

2 tablespoons melted butter.

Half a tablespoon lemon juice

Use ranch or blue cheese dressing for serving.

Use carrot and celery sticks for serving.

DIRECTIONS

1. Preheat the oven to 450° Fahrenheit. Coat a baking sheet with cooking spray or line it with parchment paper.
2. In a large mixing basin, combine flour, water, garlic powder, paprika, salt, and pepper until the batter is smooth. Toss cauliflower into the batter until coated.
3. Spread cauliflower in a single layer on the prepared baking sheet, leaving space between them. Bake until lightly browned, about 20 to 25 minutes, flipping halfway through.
4. In a separate small bowl, add the spicy sauce, melted butter, and lemon juice until thoroughly combined. Brush the cauliflower with the buffalo sauce mixture.
5. Return to the oven for approximately 15 minutes, or until they begin to brown.
6. Serve hot with ranch dressing, celery, and carrots, if desired.

109

DESSERTS

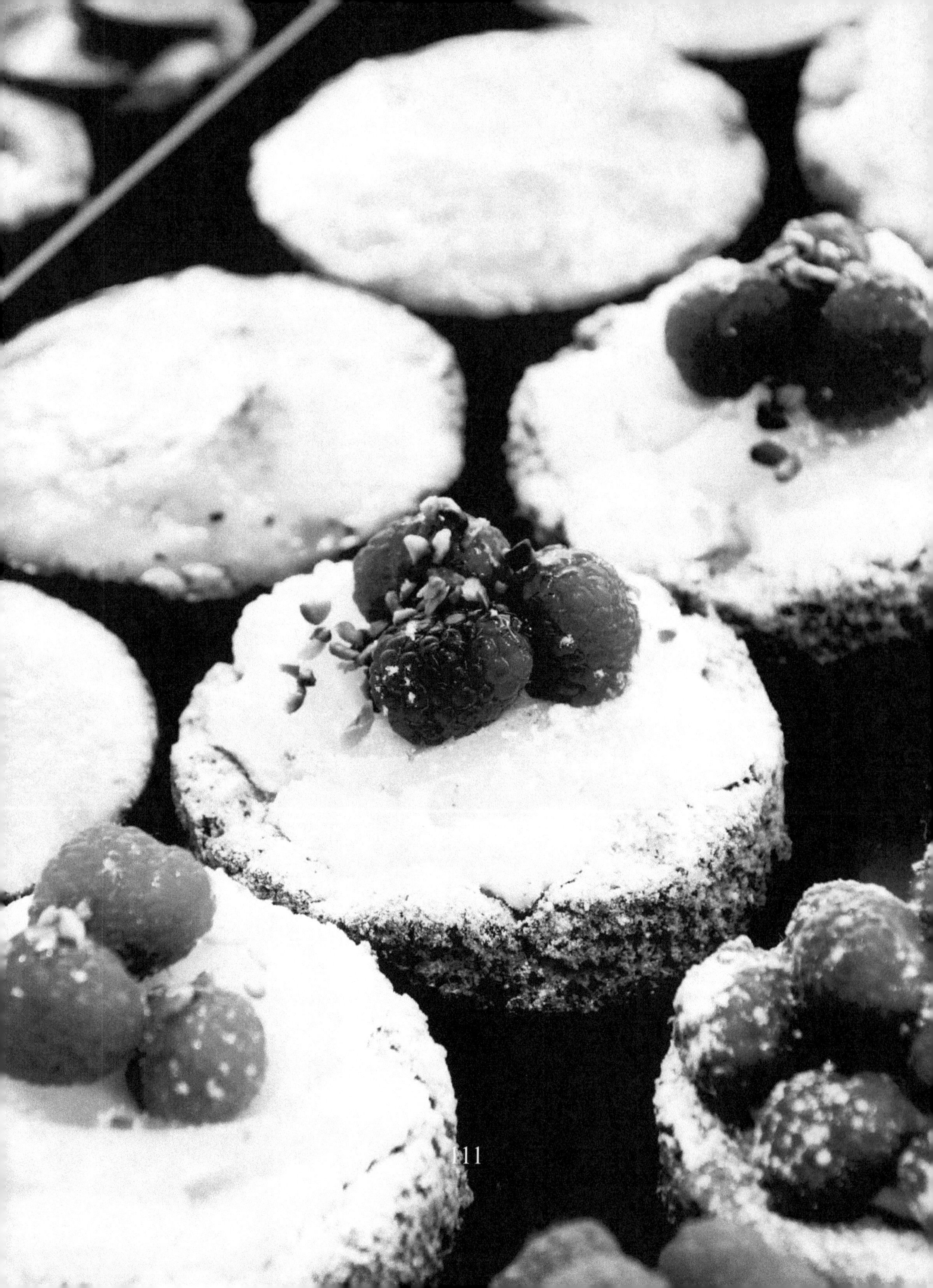

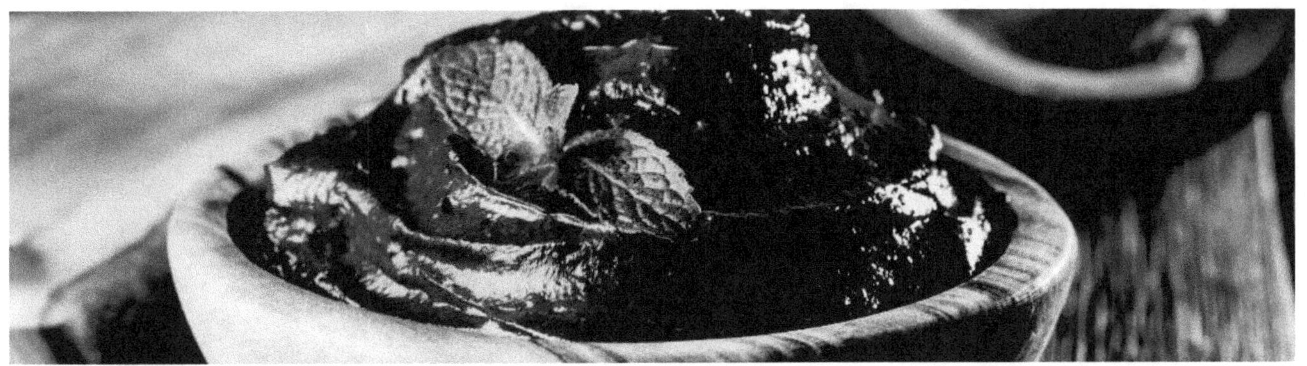

Dark chocolate avocado mousse

CALORIES: 497   **FAT: 31G**   **PROTEIN: 4.5G**   **CARB: 50G**

SERVINGS: 4   **PREP TIME: 10 MINS**   **COOK TIME: 40 MINS**

INGREDIENTS

Two really ripe avocados.
4 ounces 70% cacao baking chocolate, melted*
1/4 cup unsweetened cocoa powder.
1/3 cup almond milk.
1/3 cup maple syrup.
1/2 teaspoon of vanilla extract.
1/4 teaspoon ground cinnamon, sea salt.
Optional toppings include chocolate whipped cream or coconut whipped cream, roughly chopped dark chocolate, berries, almonds, and more.

DIRECTIONS

1. In a food processor, mix together the avocados, melted chocolate, cocoa powder, maple syrup, almond milk, vanilla, cinnamon, and a touch of salt. Puree until creamy. Place the mousse in four tiny ramekins and chill for at least one hour.
2. Serve the mousse with a dollop of whipped cream and/or any desired toppings

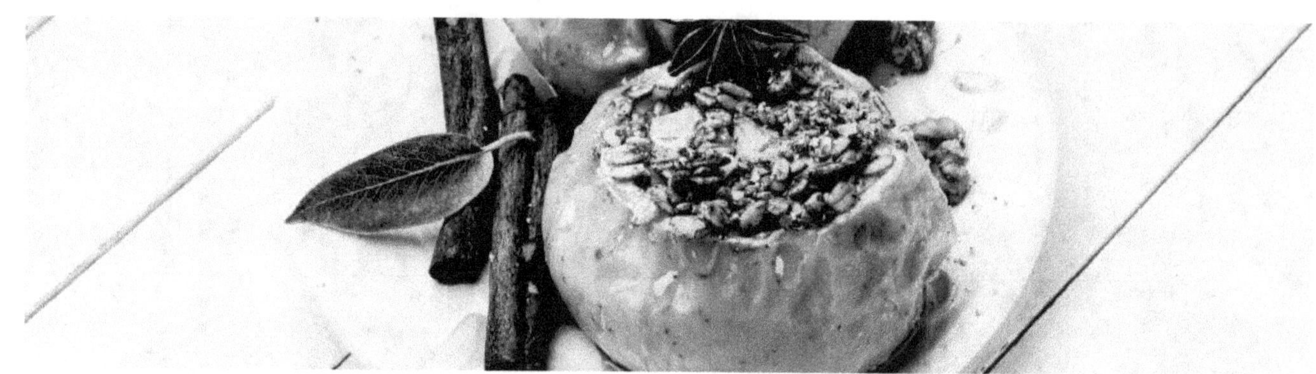

Baked apples with cinnamon and walnuts

CALORIES: 248   **FAT: 9G**   **PROTEIN: 2G**   **CARB: 41G**

SERVINGS: 4   **PREP TIME: 10 MINS**   **COOK TIME: 20 MINS**

INGREDIENTS

Four huge apples.

¼ cup maple syrup

1/2 cup chopped walnuts.

1 teaspoon of vanilla extract.

1 teaspoon of cinnamon.

DIRECTIONS

1. Preheat the oven to 350°F (175°C).
2. In a medium bowl, combine maple syrup, chopped walnuts, vanilla, and cinnamon. Allow the filling to settle while you core the apples.
3. Core four entire apples, leaving the bottoms intact. This keeps the contents from pouring out.
4. Place the apples in a baking dish and evenly distribute the prepared walnut filling.
5. Bake for twenty minutes. After 20 minutes of baking, the apples should be tender yet somewhat crisp in the center. If you want them perfectly soft, continue baking for another 10 minutes or more.
6. Serve warm, topped with chopped walnuts, maple syrup or honey, and a sprinkle of cinnamon.

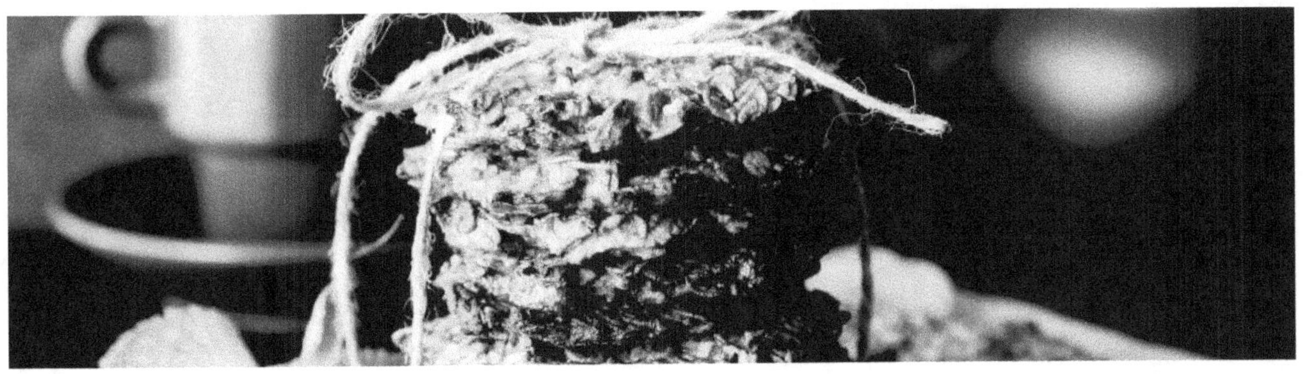

Banana Oatmeal Cookies

CALORIES: 158   **FAT: 5G**   **PROTEIN: 2G**   **CARB: 25G**

SERVINGS: 7   **PREP TIME: 15 MINS**   **COOK TIME: 15 MINS**

INGREDIENTS

1 medium-sized peeled banana

1 2 tbsp honey

1 tbsp soft or melted coconut oil

50 g (1/2 cup) rolled oats (if
gluten-free) If using chocolate
chips, ensure they are gluten-free.
Add a touch of salt.

DIRECTIONS

1. Preheat the oven to 170C/325F (fan).
2. Place the banana in a medium-sized basin and mash with a fork. Add the oats, honey, and coconut oil, and whisk well to blend. Allow to sit on the counter for 10 minutes so that the oats can absorb the moisture from the other ingredients.
3. After 10 minutes, stir in the chocolate chips (save a few to sprinkle on top once the cookies are done) and salt. Stir to mix.
4. Take a tbsp of the mixture and roll it into a ball before squashing it to form a thick disk (about 1cm thick). Place on a baking tray and repeat until all of the mixture has been used.
5. Place in the oven for 15 minutes.
6. Take out of the oven, sprinkle with the reserved chocolate chips, and let cool.

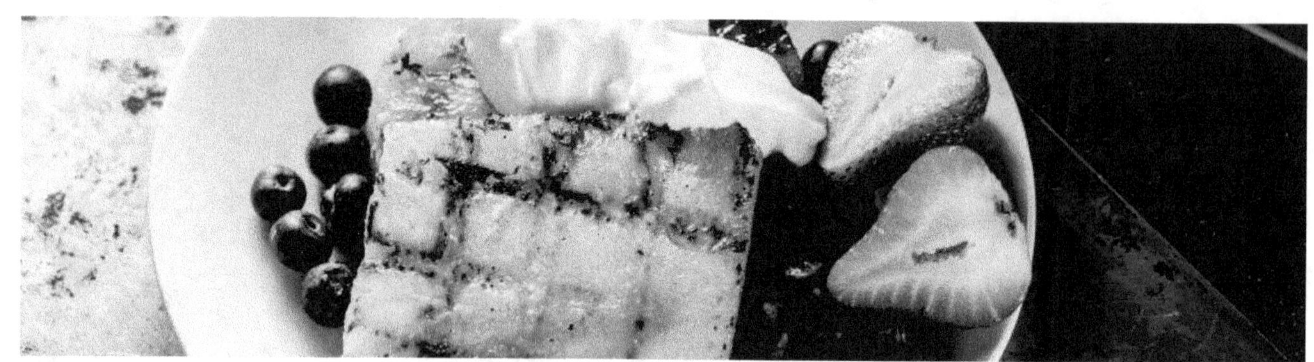

Grilled pineapple with honey and Greek yogurt

SERVINGS: 4 **PREP TIME: 10 MINS** **COOK TIME: 5 MINS**

INGREDIENTS

One pineapple, sliced into rounds.

1/2 cup Greek yogurt.

2 tablespoons of honey.

Add 2 teaspoons of cinnamon and decorate with mint sprigs.

DIRECTIONS

1. Heat the grill or grill pan, then lightly oil it. Put on the pineapple slices and cook for about 2-3 minutes, or until grill marks emerge. Flip and cook for another 2-3 minutes.
2. In a bowl, combine Greek yogurt, honey, and cinnamon.
3. To serve, stack two pieces of pineapple (or more if desired) on top of each other, followed by a generous serving of Greek yogurt. If desired, sprinkle more cinnamon on top. Garnish with mint sprigs.

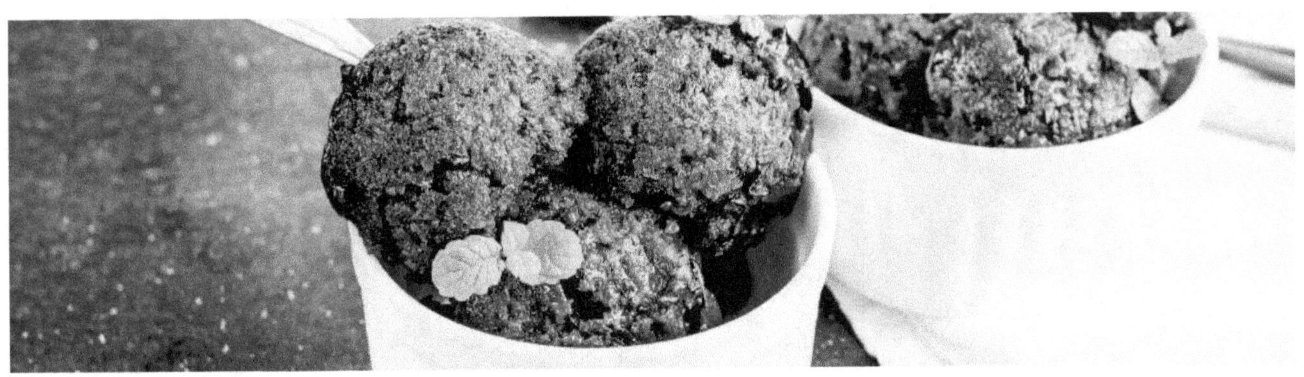

Berry Sorbet with Mint

CALORIES: 131   **FAT: 0.4G**   **PROTEIN: 1G**   **CARB: 33G**

SERVINGS: 8   **PREP TIME: 10 MINS**   **COOK TIME: 15 MINS**

INGREDIENTS

500 g raspberries (~4 cups), plus
a few more for garnish.
200 g granulated sugar (about 1
cup)
3/4 cup water.
2 tablespoons fresh lemon juice
5 g mint (approximately 2 loose
tablespoons), plus a few leaves
for garnish.

DIRECTIONS

1. Place the raspberries and sugar in a large, non-reactive basin and refrigerate overnight. If you're short on time, simply combine the ingredients and set them on the counter for around 30 minutes.
2. Put the fruit/sugar combination and the additional ingredients in a blender and purée until smooth. If your blender isn't very powerful, you may wish to pre-mince the mint.
3. Pour and push the mixture through a mesh or fine strainer to remove the majority of the seeds. Discard the seeds.
4. Chill the sorbet mixture in the refrigerator for at least two hours.
5. Add the cool sorbet mixture to an ice cream machine and freeze according to the manufacturer's directions.
6. Store the completed sorbet in the freezer. Allow around 1 hour for a softer, looser sorbet. Allow sorbet to freeze for 4-5 hours or overnight.

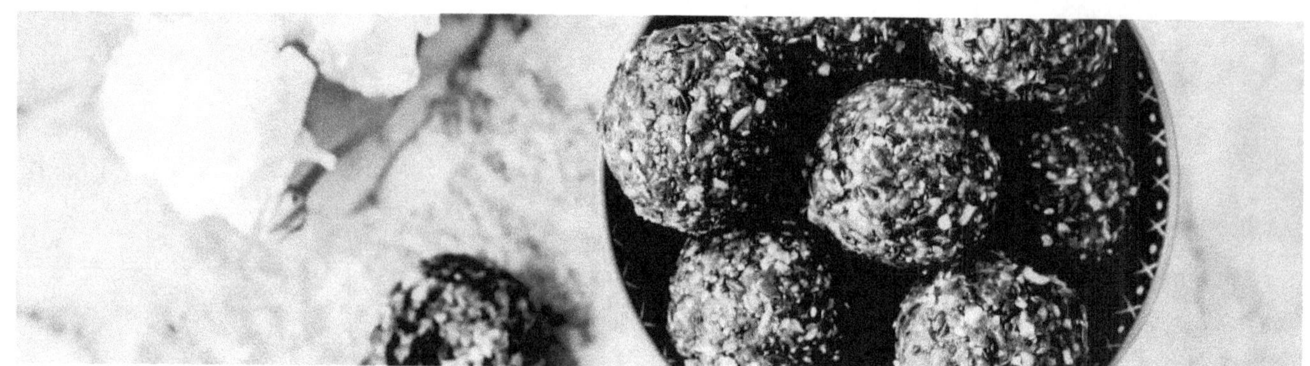

Almond Butter Energy Balls

CALORIES: 181   **FAT: 12.1G**   **PROTEIN: 4.7G**   **CARB: 17.4G**

SERVINGS: 4   **PREP TIME: 10 MINS**   **TOTAL TIME: 20 MINS**

INGREDIENTS

⅔ cup almond butter
6 tablespoons brown rice syrup
(or maple syrup)
1 cup old-fashioned rolled oats,
½ cup flaxseed meal
½ cup vegan dark chocolate.
1/2 teaspoon vanilla extract
1-2 tablespoons water (if dough
is too dry)
¼ teaspoon sea salt

DIRECTIONS

1. In a mixing bowl, blend fresh drippy almond butter, brown rice syrup, and, if desired, vanilla extract until thick and creamy.
2. Stir in the oats, ground flaxseed, and salt, if desired. The mixture is difficult to stir, so lubricate your hands with coconut oil and knead and squeeze it. If it's too dry, add 1-2 more tablespoons of water.
3. Fold in the chocolate chips and mix until combined.
4. Refrigerate the bowl for 10-15 minutes to make the batter easier to roll into energy balls and allow the fiber to absorb the liquid.
5. Meanwhile, cover a dish with parchment paper. Set it away.
6. Remove the bowl from the refrigerator. Lightly grease your hands with coconut oil, then roll roughly 1-2 tablespoons of batter between them.
7. Place each energy bite on the prepared dish, and repeat until all of the batter has been converted into bliss balls.

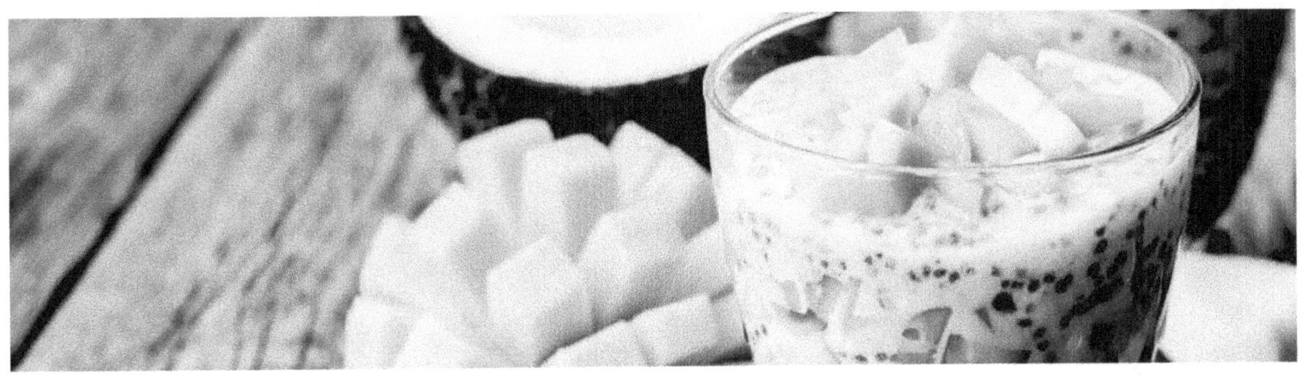

Coconut Yogurt with Mango Cubes

CALORIES: 210　　**FAT: 2G**　　**PROTEIN: 6G**　　**CARB: 25G**

SERVINGS: 4　　**PREP TIME: 10 MINS**　　**COOK TIME: 10 MINS**

INGREDIENTS

2 mangos.

4 Amaretti cookies (about 1.5 ounces each)

Two small containers of coconut yogurt (5.3 ounces each)

DIRECTIONS

1. Peel mangos and chop meat into ½ inch cubes.
2. Use your fingers to break the cookies into little pieces.
3. Pour 1 tablespoon yogurt into each shot glass.
4. Top with 1 T mango cubes and 1/2 T amaretto cookie crumbles.
5. Repeat with another layer similar to the first, ending with cookie crumbles.

Conclusion

In "Healthy Diet for Sleep Disorders," we looked at how dietary choices can have a significant impact on sleep quality and overall health. Individuals can improve their sleep hygiene by eating a well-balanced diet rich in nutrient-dense foods including whole grains, lean meats, fruits, vegetables, and healthy fats.

Throughout this book, we've looked at the science behind how specific nutrients and dietary patterns affect sleep, from promoting relaxation to regulating neurotransmitters required for the sleep-wake cycle. We've highlighted practical techniques for incorporating these nutrients into regular meals, allowing readers to make informed decisions that help them achieve their sleep goals.

It's critical to understand that getting enough sleep is more than simply what we eat; it's also about developing good lifestyle habits like regular exercise, stress management, and creating a suitable sleep environment. By incorporating these strategies into our everyday routines, we can develop a more comprehensive approach to sleep wellness.

Remember that everyone's journey to improved sleep is unique, and it may take some testing and modifications to figure out what works best for them. With devotion and the knowledge learned from this book, you will be able to go on a path to increased sleep quality, better overall health, and a more vibrant existence.

Here's to sustaining your body, mind, and soul with the power of nutritious food and adequate sleep.

I HAVE REQUEST

Dear Readers,

I hope you found "Healthy Diet for Sleep Disorders" informative and useful in your path to better sleep and general health. Your feedback means a lot to me, and it can help others discover how this book might improve their lives.

Would you please consider leaving a review whether it's about what you loved best, how the book helped you, or recommendations for improvement, it will be very appreciated.

Thank you so much for your encouragement and for being a part of this path to better sleep patterns.

Warm regards.

Sonia Cline

www.ingramcontent.com/pod-product-compliance
Lightning Source LLC
Chambersburg PA
CBHW081649260726
48653CB00009BA/3321